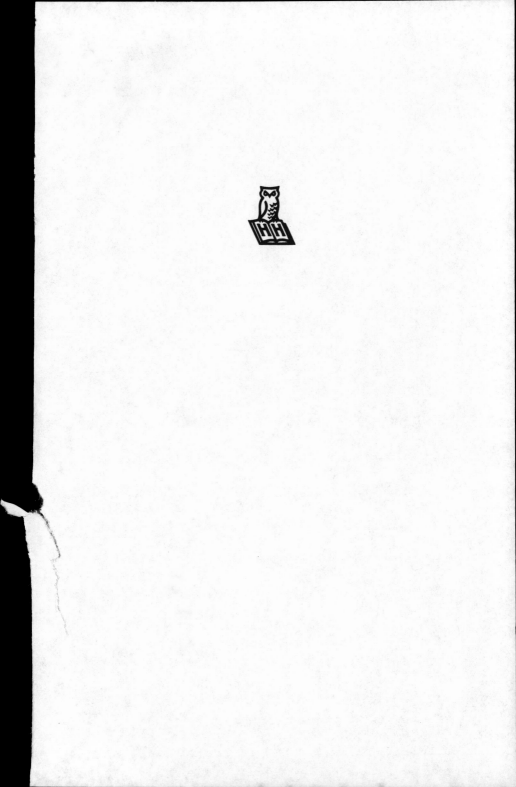

# AN
# UNSPOKEN ART

# AN
# UNSPOKEN ART

## Profiles of Veterinary Life

## Lee Gutkind

HENRY HOLT AND COMPANY
NEW YORK

Henry Holt and Company, Inc.
*Publishers since 1866*
115 West 18th Street
New York, New York 10011

Henry Holt® is a registered trademark of
Henry Holt and Company, Inc.

Library of Congress Cataloging-in-Publication Data
Gutkind, Lee.
An unspoken art: profiles of veterinary life / Lee Gutkind.—1st ed.
p.  cm.
"Portions of this book were first published in slightly different forms in Prairie
schooner, The Sonora review, and The crab orchard review and in The art of
nonfiction: writing and selling the literature of reality, published by John Wiley &
Sons"—T.p. verso.
Includes index.
 1. Veterinarians—United States.  2. Veterinary  medicine—United States.
3. Veterinary medicine—Vocational guidance—United States.  4. Veterinarians.
5. Veterinary  medicine.  6.  Veterinary  medicine—Vocational  guidance.
I. Title.
SF623.G88   1997                                              96-29503
636.089'092'273—dc21                                              CIP

ISBN 0-8050-3321-1

Henry Holt books are available for special promotions and premiums.
For details contact: Director, Special Markets.

First Edition—1997

Designed by Jessica Shatan

Printed in the United States of America
All first editions are printed on acid-free paper. ∞

1  3  5  7  9  10  8  6  4  2

Portions of this book were first published in slightly different forms in *Prairie
Schooner, The Sonora Review,* and *The Crab Orchard Review* and in *The Art of
Nonfiction: Writing and Selling the Literature of Reality,* published by John Wiley &
Sons. Reprinted by permission.

*To my lifelong friends,*

*dedicated animal lovers Bob and Susan Simon*

# CONTENTS

# ACKNOWLEDGMENTS

I wish to express appreciation to the University of Pennsylvania's School of Veterinary Medicine, the Pittsburgh Zoo, the Center for Veterinary Care for opening their facilities to me, and to Helma Weeks and Michael Hennessy, DVM, for their insight and consultation. Patricia Park, my boon companion for many years, contributed her always reliable commentary, while Nancy Brown's copyediting and M. A. Sinnuber's transcribing were invaluable. Thanks also to my editors, William Strachan, for his continued faith and support, and Darcy Tromanhauser, for her steadfast feedback.

# AN
# UNSPOKEN ART

# INTRODUCTION

# "We Lay Our Hands Down upon Them"

·————————————————·

This was to be my fourth exploration of a medical community—preceded by books about organ transplant surgeons, pediatric hospitals, and children with mental health problems. But I soon learned that medicine is only part of what veterinarians are all about. Veterinarians are primarily interested in biology, ecology, and the natural world—all things that must be nurtured to live and grow. They also possess a particularly focused concept of the lifestyle they want to lead. By necessity, they are much more people-oriented and humanistic than the vast majority of physicians about whom I have written.

Consider, for example, the prototypical veterinary model, Scottish-born James Alfred Wight, who was inspired as an adolescent by an article in a magazine that dramatized veterinary life. Urbane and cultured, Wight's parents were renowned classical musicians. But after graduating Glasgow Veterinary College,

Introduction

Wight's first veterinary position treating farm animals in an isolated rural area of Yorkshire Dales in northern England would
last more than fifty years, a delightful surprise, he once said. "I
hadn't thought it possible that I could spend all my days in a
high, clean blown land where the scent of grass or trees was
never far away, and where, even in the driving rain of winter, I
could sniff the air and find the freshness of growing things hid-
den somewhere in the cold clasp of the wind. . . . I was a
privileged person."

Like Wight, most of the veterinarians about whom I write in
this book were affected by the concept of a fulfilling and "privileged" lifestyle, beginning at a very early age. Arthur Bramson,
born and raised in East Flatbush in Brooklyn, was inspired by an
experience in the country when he was eight years old. Bramson
always loved animals, but he remembers walking down a quiet
road in the middle of the summer with his parents and passing a
farm where a cow was giving birth to a calf, aided by a veterinarian. He watched breathlessly. "After that, there was nothing else
I ever wanted to be," he said.

Gene Solomon, who practices in Manhattan's Upper East
Side, became a veterinarian because of the company he found in
animals. Solomon's father died before he was born, and his
mother, who never remarried, dedicated her life to raising her
three children. Solomon found support and comfort with animals, especially those who, like himself, lacked a parent or family. "From when I was five years old, I was bringing stray animals
home."

Wendy Freeman grew up on a small farm with cattle, chickens, horses, the family dog, and the barn cats. "The big treat for
us kids was when the vet came to work on one of the animals;
we'd sit and watch. I saw calves being born when I was very
small; it inspired me."

Horses inspired Wendy Vaala. Born and raised in the suburbs

2

near Wilmington, Delaware, Vaala adopted the neighborhood's orphaned animals, filling house and yard with dogs, cats, rabbits, and wounded birds. Eventually, she talked her parents into providing riding lessons, and "I just kept nagging until I got a horse of my own in the fifth grade."

During her senior year in high school, Vaala visited the University of Pennsylvania's large animal hospital, New Bolton Center, near Kennett Square in Chester County, to research a report—and immediately signed on for a five-week summer internship. Vaala attended Penn as an undergraduate and four years of veterinary school, concluding with an internship at New Bolton—back where she started. Except for a brief year in private practice, Vaala never left New Bolton. Today, as founder and director of the high-risk pregnancy program in the Neonatal Intensive Care Unit there, she works with many of the professors who originally taught her.

Vaala's colleague, Patricia Sertich, although equally passionate about the profession, was initially not as self-directed. Sertich grew up in coal mining country. As an undergraduate at West Virginia University, Sertich intended to enter pharmacy school until she learned in her first semester that "pharmacy" and "farm" were significantly different. She changed her major to animal science, then earned a graduate degree in reproductive physiology and endocrinology before entering veterinary school. Today she is the gynecologist for the mares in Vaala's high-risk pregnancy program in the New Bolton ICU.

"I have a horse that's thirty-two years old," Sertich told me, "and I joke that he's the reason I'm a veterinarian, because I wanted to make him live forever. At home, I have six horses. I've had horses all my life. Here, I work all day with horses, I go home, and the first thing I do is go for a horseback ride."

Veterinarians and their clients share all-consuming and often frustrating eccentricities concerning the care and treatment of their animals, a fact that repeatedly amazed James Alfred Wight. A consummate storyteller who delighted family and friends with anecdotes about the animals he treated and their owners, Wight kept a journal in which details of his cases were recorded over nearly three decades. When he was fifty-three, he bought an old typewriter and set it up in a back room to begin converting his notes into stories, a process that he found to be slow-going and lonely. Missing the company of his wife and children, he eventually moved his "office" into the family room, where he could also keep tabs on the soccer season on television. Simultaneously cheering and writing, he was so enthused by a game one day he decided to adopt as a pen name the last name of his favorite goalie. Thus, "James Herriot" was created just before the publication of Wight's first major book, *All Creatures Great and Small*. Over the next quarter-century, that title and Wight's sixteen subsequent books (*All Creatures Bright and Beautiful*, etc.)—aided by a feature film and a long-running BBC television series—would sell more than sixty million copies.

While subtly demonstrating high-quality basic veterinary medicine, Herriot's books are quite ethnographic, humorously capturing the superstitions and eccentricities of his farmer-clients. Herriot, although a traditionalist in many ways, valued technology; from the beginning, his dream of becoming a veterinarian always included the most up-to-date medications and a laboratory with modern equipment. Indeed, there are today a small number of veterinarians primarily in cutting-edge academic settings who can do almost as much for their patients from a technological standpoint as can doctors in the most advanced human medical facilities. But as veterinarians soon discover, sophisticated diagnostic tools are often useless in the muck, mud, and isolation of a farm, a zoo, or an exotic wildlife practice; flexibility and adaptability, however, are always crucial. Among many impressive procedures at the Pittsburgh Zoo, I observed veterinarians remove a tusk (a "tuskectomy") from an elephant in danger of dying from neurological impairment caused by an infected tooth, using a monkey wrench, a power drill, a chisel, and a crowbar. I observed two young veterinarians operating *on their knees*, literally, for three hours, nonstop, utilizing ropes, cardboard boxes, hoists, extension cords, and other contraptions to remove an umbilical hernia with an abscess from a North American reindeer in an unlit, unheated stable.

My observation that veterinarians seem more people-oriented and humanistic than many physicians is not meant to be demeaning to physicians, but to underscore the difficulty of communicating with a nonhuman species, especially when it is frightened, sick, and in pain. In the treatment of human adults, it is assumed that doctors will speak directly with patients; and while a parent or guardian must interpret, ask questions, and make decisions for infants and toddlers, as children mature, they can more easily answer questions concerning pain, discomfort, pleasure. But no matter how mature, an animal will seldom respond reliably; in fact, the natural instinct of survival in the wild is to mask pain and handicap, which can turn the most routine diagnosis into complicated detective work. With few exceptions, veterinarians lack the sophisticated technological tools of the medical doctor (CT Scan, MRI, etc.) to aid and confirm diagnosis, relying instead on basic textbook diagnostic skills and their ability to unearth details through a focused medical history. In this day and age in which the health care world is becoming increasingly dehumanized, veterinarians spend more time and invest more energy communing with animals and worried owners than physicians with human patients.

The most noticeable difference between the way in which a veterinarian communicates with an animal and a medical doctor with a human patient is in the realm of direct physical contact. I am talking about touch—the laying on of hands—a soothing gesture that repeatedly proves therapeutic to animals, at least in a psychological sense. As I delved into the world of veterinary medicine, I found myself wishing that sick people who went to doctors were treated like animals; that is, that humans were touched in a special caring way by their doctors, looked in the eye and talked to with interest and compassion, as most veterinarians will do with their patients.

For my book about organ transplantation, I was initially enticed by the potential of transplantation to save lives. What began to affect me, though, was the pain and suffering organ transplantation (and other forms of high-tech medicine for critically ill patients) caused, not only to patients, but to the families who had to support them through surgery and recovery—and far beyond. But what also struck me then and continues to affect me now years later is the basic dearth of compassion—that vital human touch. Not only does the technology (medications, machinery, computerization) eliminate a large measure of human contact, but it also serves seemingly to deny the necessity for or expectations of courtesy and compassion.

On the organ transplant service, I remember listening to a prominent surgeon interrupting a resident explaining a procedure to a family member by imploring him to "save lives first—answer questions later." Another surgeon told me, in defense of his insensitive behavior, "Psychologic trauma and all that stuff is important, but it doesn't make a goddamn difference if you are well-adjusted and dead." Saving lives of dying patients becomes a surgeon's obsession, but in the process, such a single-minded and narrow pursuit seems to alter or destroy their sense of purpose—the reasons they endured years of medical training and took the Hippocratic oath.

I never felt that way about veterinarians during all the time I researched and wrote this book. Here were men and women, obviously interested in lifesaving, but dedicated and devoted to the psychological well-being of their patients. This is the missing link in human medicine: Many of our caregivers do not regard or treat their patients as human beings.

And this is the part of veterinary medicine I will never forget, that part that includes philosopher Erich Fromm's observation that humankind "is biologically endowed with the capacity for biophilia, the passionate love of life and all that is alive"—and the way in which it is exemplified in veterinary medicine—by human contact, by touching.

In this book, you will observe Lisa, a young veterinary technician at the Center for Veterinary Care in Manhattan, squatting uncomfortably for hours in a cramped cage and in pools of urine, cooing over and petting a dying West Highland terrier named Annabelle; a zoo veterinarian, Steven Marks, who stays awake, night after night, in the living room of his home desperately attempting to preserve the life of a baby bongo in a jerry-rigged cage in his kitchen; and many other passionate and sacrificial acts of caring.

I was lucky to witness a revolutionary cryosurgical technique at New Bolton on a prized racehorse named Cam Fella. The procedure was incredibly exciting, but the most memorable part of the experience occurred long after the surgery, long after the owners had departed and most of the entourage and the curious onlookers had disappeared. Eight exhausted veterinarians and nurses, all women, remained in the recovery area with Cam Fella, sitting in a circle, elbow-to-elbow, keeping him calm. Touching him. Kissing him. Talking to him. Until he was awake enough to stand on his own and navigate the winding path back to his stall.

Veterinarians feel that they owe their patients this special quality of attention. It is a vital and unavoidable lesson that human doctors must learn. "We do everything possible to make an animal psychologically and physiologically happy after the physical and emotional strain of the experience. We lay our hands down upon them," veterinary anesthesiologist Kim Olsen told me. This is certainly the least—and perhaps the very most—all doctors can do. It is what Manhattan veterinarian Amy Attas describes as "God's work"—and it is the work veterinarians do each day.

# DOING "GOD'S WORK"

·——————————————————————————————·

O riginally, Amy Attas, a Manhattan veterinarian who had graduated from the University of Pennsylvania's School of Veterinary Medicine five years before, had assumed that she and her employer, a prominent Park Avenue veterinarian, would one day become partners. He had frequently encouraged the partnership prospect, but on the day they were scheduled to meet for an annual salary review—they had made plans to go out for a drink after the meeting—he called Attas into his office and abruptly fired her.

Attas was stunned. And, fearful that being dismissed in such a cursory and mysterious manner made it appear as if she had committed a crime or violated scientific or ethical veterinary principles, she hired a labor lawyer and sued her former boss, who was maintaining that Attas had not been performing in a satisfactory manner. But after a long wait, followed by a trial lasting three weeks, a jury reached a verdict in Attas's favor, awarding her more than $400,000. Amy Attas's reputation, not to mention her bank account, had been safeguarded.

Long before the Attas jury had reached its verdict, however, long before the case had even gone to court, Amy Attas realized that her former employer had inadvertently created for her the opportunity of a lifetime. The morning after being fired, Attas received a phone call from a client with a sick animal. She explained that she no longer had an office to treat patients, but the client was insistent, so Attas decided to visit the woman and the dog at home. From that point on, Amy Attas's business started to grow. She became a house-call veterinarian, perhaps the most successful and certainly the most prominent of the few hundred full-time house-call veterinarians in the world.

The lawsuit Attas filed against her former boss and the firing that precipitated it are not typical of the veterinary community in the United States. In Manhattan, however, with probably more veterinarians per city block than in any other large urban area, as well as the highest fees for veterinary services in the world, competition is fierce. And nationally, veterinary medicine is undergoing a gender change that is having a significant impact on the old-boy power structure, traditionally the dominating force of the profession. Two decades ago, fewer than five of one hundred graduate doctors of veterinary medicine were women. In 1935, there were only five female veterinarians in the entire country. Today, seven of ten students gaining admission to veterinary schools are women, thus signaling a new and important trend.

There are different schools of thought surrounding the sudden influx of women. A justification for excluding women in the past was because women were considered physically incapable of controlling large farm animals such as cows and horses, but today, such theories are brushed aside by men and women alike. In fact, the smaller size of women's hands may be more suitable for animal work.

Besides, small animal practices (dogs, cats, birds, etc.) in which women have been most comfortable, today dominate the profession. According to a recent survey by the American Pet Products Manufacturers Association, 56 percent of all Americans own a pet. The average pet owner is married, lives in a house (as opposed to an apartment or condominium), is under fifty years old, and does not have children living with them. Among dog and cat owners, the average number of pets per household is nearly two; the number increases to almost three among bird, small animal, and fish owners. Not all animal owners will consult veterinarians on a regular basis, but veterinarians in a variety of capacities will have contact with most animals in any given year. The majority of dog and cat owners will visit a veterinarian at least once annually.

Battle of the sexes aside, Attas profoundly appreciates the rewards of the veterinary profession and her specific role as a doctor who treats animals and their owners from both a physical and emotional perspective. "If you're one of the unlucky people who have to work for a living, there is no greater job than what I'm doing," she told me. "I take care of dogs and cats. My goal is to relieve them from whatever suffering they have. It's like doing 'God's Work.'"

She is referring to the fact that many clients have established a unique intimacy with animals and veterinarians. People are often frightened and panicked when their pets are sick. She is available to help talk them through a crisis—or come to their aid. "I do a lot of triage on the telephone.

"My beeper goes off at night. It goes off when I'm at the opera. It goes off on Saturdays, Sundays, and holidays. My work is much more time-consuming than most other people's, but also more rewarding. People trust me. In fact, people consult me about their own health problems. I'll go into people's homes, and a woman will lift up her blouse, show me a mole and say, 'Do you have any idea what this is?' One of my clients called one night quite late. She said, 'My daughter has head lice. I'm embarrassed to call the family physician. I knew I could turn to you for help.'

"Another client said to us one day," referring to Arthur Carter, the publisher of the New York Observer, " 'Montana is the only person allowed to eat off of my plate.' Now there are two odd things there. The first is, Montana is not a person, he's a cat. And the second is, I wouldn't let an animal eat off my plate. I really don't want anybody to eat off my plate, except maybe my husband. So the significance of the animal in this very important and intelligent man's life is really amazing." But in this regard, Arthur Carter is not unique.

I once accompanied Amy Attas to Arthur Carter's sumptuous apartment. Attas is a walking encyclopedia of East Side pets and the posh apartment buildings they live in. As we drove to the Carter home, she said: "Look at all these buildings. I can tell you about all the pets in each of them. I know the dogs who are friendly and the cats who are not." (Recently, a frightened cat bit her hand during treatment, an incident that rendered her incapable of doing surgery for five months.) Attas receives eighty dollars per house call (perhaps 25 percent higher than the average Manhattan veterinary hospital rates) and approximately two hundred dollars for a chemotherapy treatment, depending on the drug-treatment protocol being used. Cancer is a big part of her practice; six golden retrievers in the past two weeks had been diagnosed with the disease.

As we walked down the hall toward Montana Carter's bedroom, we passed the exercise room. Mr. Carter was on the treadmill. "For a long time he wouldn't acknowledge the fact that Montana was sick—and getting sicker." At that point, Montana, normally a twelve-pound cat, weighed only six pounds. "I said, 'Mr. Carter, this is cancer. And if you continue to delude yourself, the cat's going to die very soon.' "

After accepting Attas's diagnosis, Carter decided to put Montana to sleep. He had seen too many people suffer through chemotherapy; he did not want his pet to undergo such trauma—until Attas explained the vital distinction in approach to treatment between pets and people. "Our goal with chemotherapy in humans is to kill as much of the cancer as possible, even if we come very close to killing the patient in the process. But pets don't live that long. You can't explain to a cat that they will feel better later if they suffer now." Veterinarians attempt to extend life quality through chemotherapy without the promise of saving a life. "For pets, in the end," said Attas, "the cancer always wins." Attas assured Carter that Montana could be treated and proposed that she come once a week and administer the chemotherapy to Montana at home, in his own room. Carter agreed, but balked at administering the steroid twice daily as required with chemotherapy. George, the veterinary technician who works with Attas, thus visited Montana at 8:00 A.M. and 5:00 P.M., seven days a week to give prednisone. Montana went into remission; he lived comfortably for a year and a half longer.

Carter was so appreciative of Attas's service and her straightforward and intimate manner that he began recommending Amy Attas to his famous friends and colleagues who owned pets. Attas's client list includes the extended members of the Kennedy clan, who have become her friends. "I was a guest at the Kennedy Palm Beach house for a week. It was really an experience, just to sit in the chair that President Kennedy sat in." Another client, comedian Joan Rivers, has been equally influential in Attas's success by recommending Attas to all of her pet-owning friends.

Meanwhile, talking nonstop to Montana, George chased the

cat around the antique chests and majestic four-poster bed. "You know, we don't actually expect Montana or any other cat to understand or talk back to us when we talk to them," he told me.

"We don't?" asked Attas.

George laughed. "This sounds like a recent conversation I had with my shrink. I told him: 'Even though I constantly talk to my cats, I realize they don't understand what I am saying.'

"And my shrink said, 'They don't?'

" 'Well, no,' I said.

" 'That's funny,' my shrink replied. 'Mine do.' "

Although there are significant cultural differences from place to place in this country and abroad, people who love animals are very much the same. There are more than a few Arthur Carters outside Manhattan—owners willing to allocate mountains of money to the care and treatment of a cat. And there are many thousands willing to invest as much or more in a beloved horse—or pig, parrot, or goat. They invest what they can afford—and often much more—in the health and well-being of their animals, for whom they frequently display a deep and unwavering devotion. There are those who might object to money "squandered" on pets, while ignoring the wealth invested in Mercedes-Benz cars, diamond brooches, Las Vegas gambling, and travel—considerably less worthy endeavors than animal ownership, which has existed nearly as long as man has lived in civilized society.

When a dog died in ancient Egypt, owners and their families shaved themselves as an expression of mourning. The Egyptians also venerated their cats—and embalmed them. A visitor can view a mummified cat at the University of Pennsylvania's museum, its wizened face illuminated behind mysterious layers of shrouds. There is something very basic and ethereal about an appreciation of pets and a love for animals in this society—an experience that offers a universal lesson in boundless compassion.

Humankind, according to the psychologist Erich Fromm, "is biologically endowed with the capacity for biophilia," which is the "passionate love of life and all that is alive." If Fromm is correct, says Elizabeth Atwood Lawrence, who is both a veterinarian and a cultural anthropologist, then love for animals is more than a frivolous emotion possessed by a certain group of people, such as veterinarians. "Rather, it is a natural manifestation of what it means to be human—a quality that not only enhances our species' well-being, but may be vital to the health and preservation of the planet. . . . Veterinarians, in their role of mediating between human beings and the animal world, are in a unique position to foster and facilitate the expression of biophilia."

"About a dozen years ago," said Amy Attas, "when I was a veterinary student, I saw a little pug dog tied to a tree. There was a note attached to the tree which said, 'I am blind. Please take good care of me.'

"I could not believe that someone had abandoned this little pug. So I took him inside the hospital. He was skinny. He was flea-ridden. I mean, he was a mess. I brought him upstairs. I bathed him. I vaccinated him. I put him in a cage, and I said, 'Listen, kid, I don't want a dog. Tomorrow, I'll take you to the pound. But just to be nice, you can have a home-cooked meal at my house tonight.' Then I went to work.

"He's totally blind, remember. But every time I went past his cage, he would recognize my smell and jump and bark. The rest of the time, he would stay there looking pathetic. At the end of the day, I scooped him up, put him in the car, drove him home with me. My apartment was fairly small, but he bumped his way around every wall in every room. Then he returned to the front door, lifted his leg and peed, as if to say, 'I'm home.'

"But I was annoyed. I didn't want a dog in the first place, especially one who peed on my door. So I locked him in the kitchen, gave him a home-cooked meal, and made up my mind I was going to find him a home. Went to bed that night. In the middle of the night, he found a way out of the kitchen, came into the bedroom, jumped on the bed, laid down next to me, and went to sleep. That was it. I was hooked. I named him Bumper because he literally bumped his way wherever he went. He had the sweetest disposition. He was one of the nicest dogs I ever met.

"And later when I went into practice and clients wanted to put their animals to sleep prematurely, I could introduce them to Bumper. 'Your dog doesn't have to be physically perfect,' I would tell them. 'Look at how terrific Bumper is.' He was a wonderful model to illustrate that handicaps don't matter. You can love animals just as much, even if they are a little different from what you expect. And Bumper was infinitely different. He could fetch. He walked everywhere. He'd go up the steps. I'd say 'Up, up, up, up, up,' and he'd keep jumping. When Bumper got sick and lost the use of his back legs, we had a cart built, and he'd prance around in that cart, using his front legs, and his back legs would just go along for the ride. And people would come up and say, 'You're cruel. You should put that dog to sleep.'

" 'Thank you very much. But I think you should mind your own business.' You see, Bumper had no pain. He was very happy. One day, months later, he died in his sleep. Now everybody always asks, 'When are you going to get another pet?' It's sort of odd for a veterinarian to have no pets. Well, I tell them, I rescued my dog. And some time before Bumper, I rescued a cat who was with me for sixteen years. And some day, another beast will come along and need to be rescued, and I'll find it, and it will come live with me—forever."

$A$my Attas's assertion that veterinarians do "God's Work" highlights a significant difference between practitioners of animal and human medicine—and may well isolate a vital contrast between the way in which veterinarians and MDs regard their patients. As I delved into the world of veterinary medicine, I found myself wishing repeatedly that sick people who went to doctors were treated like animals—that is, that humans were touched in a special caring way by their doctors, looked in the eye, and talked to with interest and compassion, as do most veterinarians with their patients.

Touching, petting, kissing, caressing are the easier and less complicated ways in which veterinarians treat and communicate with their patients; communicating with owners of the animals is the more difficult and frustrating challenge. Veterinarians are servants of two masters, whose best interests will often conflict. Practically and morally speaking, how does a veterinarian respond when an owner's decision conflicts with the best interests of the animal about whom the decision is made? Amy Attas successfully resolved this dilemma for Arthur and Montana Carter, but such conflicts are often not so easily and peacefully resolved.

The mitigating factor in the Montana Carter case was love for the animal, whereas in many instances the veterinarian's diagnostic and treatment decisions revolve around the owner's best interests for himself. Many people compare pediatricians and veterinarians because in both cases the patient group cannot speak for itself. Although there is a certain amount of variation in the parent-child relationship, parents generally value their children, whereas value in a veterinary milieu is often deter-mined by practicality and economics—despite a veterinarian's personal feelings concerning the animal's intrinsic worth.

James Serpell, who teaches ethics to student veterinarians at the University of Pennsylvania, is a widely respected authority on the domestic animal's role in society. He described a recent case that illustrated the intricate web of conflicting interests influencing the veterinarian's ability to diagnose and treat in a compassionate and ethical fashion. A famous racehorse devel-oped a form of lameness, which was largely untreatable and very painful. The horse, owned by a consortium of people including Arab oil magnates and movie stars, was insured for millions of dollars, but could not stand properly on its hind legs.

Had it been an ordinary pet or family horse, the veterinary surgeons would have recommended euthanasia, Serpell told me. But because of the horse's value, because of pressure from the insurance company, and also because New Bolton, Penn's large animal hospital, is supposedly the cutting-edge center for equine orthopedics, they proceeded with the delicate and challenging surgical procedure, and the long and painful recovery process. But, as expected, the problem immediately recurred. A meeting took place involving the entire consortium of owners and the insurance company, and eventually it was agreed to euthanize the animal, for which most of the veterinarians at New Bolton had lobbied from the very beginning. In the end, the resources invested had been wasted, while a helpless animal had suffered needlessly.

I once witnessed one of these cutting-edge equine procedures on a horse named Cam Fella, who had developed a malignant testicular tumor. Cam Fella, the most distinguished pacer in the history of harness racing, is the most valuable breeding stallion in the world. Since retiring in 1984, the sixteen-year-old's prog-eny have amassed the highest average earnings of any standardbred or thoroughbred. Ten have won more than $1 million in races. Cam Fella stud fees generate more than $2.5 million annually.

Normally, a horse with testicular cancer would be castrated to prevent metastasis; the remaining testicle could manufacture sperm. Cam Fella, however, was a ridgling; he had only one descended testicle. Castration would save his life, but end his career, unless veterinarians could find a way to eliminate the tumor. Their solution, after weeks of consultation, was freezing the tumor away.

Cryotherapy had been used in horses before, but this time surgeons arranged for the use of a newly developed instrument called an AccuProbe, which delivers precise amounts of liquid nitrogen with pinpoint accuracy. Surgeons freeze the tumor as close as possible to the epididymis (the coiled tubes through which the sperm travel); whether Cam Fella breeds again depends on their visual assessment—and upon whether the technique is ultimately successful. Between tumor-reducing treatments, Cam Fella was bred more than one hundred times during the February-through-July breeding season, resulting in sixty-two mares in foal. At least one additional cryosurgery will follow, and it is not at all clear whether the tumor will ever really be eradicated.

Although cryotherapy and ultrasound equipment were donated, the university charged its standard rate for services, facilities, and a dozen nurses and doctors: $2,989.71. "We researched what the entire procedure might cost if this had been done on a person," said Bob Tucker, owner of Stonegate Farms in New Jersey, where Cam Fella lives: "It was at least $50,000."

This dramatic surgery was captured in a four-page photo essay in the New York Times Magazine, and for a couple of weeks the veterinarians at Penn were heroes, but letters in the Times in response to their work that criticized the allocation of resources

for a horse and the ethical decision to operate rather than cas-
trate eventually tempered their pleasure and once again illustrated the conflicts of their profession. The letter writers did not
blame veterinarians, but rather took to task both the horse's
owners for putting Cam Fella through the procedure and medical equipment manufacturers willing to donate pricey technology to treat a $2.5 million racehorse while costs in human
medical care are skyrocketing.

But the very fact that veterinarians were morally and scientifi-
cally responsible for Cam Fella, without having the overall authority to influence the animal's future significantly, presents an
unsettling scenario for a self-portrait. How can veterinarians feel
good about themselves when they are maneuvered to the side-
lines in situations that they are so often expected to control?
Serpell suggests that a study done in England illustrates the frustration and insecurity under which most veterinarians live.
"Veterinarians are at the top of all professions in terms of suicide
and alcoholism. I don't think people are sufficiently aware of just
how difficult the veterinary life really is. And particularly in this
changing climate of public opinion."

The Western world is undergoing a global shift in terms of
public attitude toward animals, whose value is literally and morally increasing—a fact that is complicating a veterinarian's ability to serve two masters. Twelve to 15 percent of the profession
is chemically impaired. Older vets drink alcohol; younger veterinarians use drugs. "No one teaches us stress management," a
veterinary student from Louisiana State University stated at a
conference on chemical abuse. "The only thing we know to do
is drink!" Another student admitted to keeping a 50cc syringe of
euthanasia fluid in her desk drawer, "just in case things got too
tough to handle."

In light of this, Amy Attas's concept of doing "God's Work"
may be an overly romantic and exaggerated notion of the veteri-

narian's role, but in reality I think most people find themselves wishing for a doctor who would treat patients with a similarly impassioned spirit and dedication, as compared to the scientific and impersonal way in which they are normally regarded by their doctors. "God's Work" also describes the rescue fantasy, as evidenced by Attas's dog Bumper, that nearly every veterinarian shares and practices to a certain degree. And more important, like Attas, and unlike most human doctors, veterinarians will take personal responsibility for their "train wrecks," administering continued support, even in their own homes, as long as necessary.

The veterinary rescue fantasy is directly related to the potential of veterinary medicine, as well as to its limitations. Given today's technological advances, much can be accomplished to save a dying animal by one committed and focused person, in marked contrast to human medicine in which the doctor is so reliant on technology and on an extended support staff and hampered by regulations, the need for permissions every step of the way, and the paralyzing fear of litigation. In animal medicine, veterinarians can be "daring" in the best sense of the word. And if their valiant rescue efforts do not succeed, veterinarians possess a unique and invaluable escape clause called "euthanasia." The ability to end life legally is perhaps the supreme privilege and the overwhelming psychic burden of performing "God's Work."

# MANHATTAN VETERINARIAN

As in Amy Attas's work with Montana Carter, "trust" is an all-important veterinary concept; veterinarians want and need desperately to be believed and trusted to do their best for patient and owner in any situation, despite how their actions and decisions may be evaluated by an outsider, uninvolved in the animal world.

Such is the case at the Center for Veterinary Care on the Upper East Side, the third largest veterinary hospital in Manhattan. On call twenty-four hours a day, medical director Gene Solomon and his partner Paul Schwartz are in the office ten hours a day, six days a week, making decisions and recommendations that radically affect a number of fragile and consumed pet owners, often by "pushing the envelope of technology," as Solomon frequently explains. Becoming best friends and partners was predestined once they both entered the University of Florida

School of Veterinary Medicine. "I'm Solomon and he's Schwartz. Seven Jews in the entire class at the University of Florida. What do you expect?" They also operate a satellite office in Scarsdale, about twenty-five miles northeast of Manhattan.

In Baltimore, where he grew up, Solomon worked as a veterinary technician through high school. After veterinary school, he was accepted into the internship program at the Animal Medical Center (AMC), the largest private animal hospital in the world, caring for 62,000 patients annually (internships are voluntary and placement is competitive in veterinary medicine). Solomon then joined Lewis Berman, a short, balding veterinarian at Park East Animal Hospital, which is on Park Avenue and 64th Street, whose practice, founded in 1963, has become the model to emulate on the Upper East Side for those veterinarians who care to cater to the rich and famous. Solomon remained with Berman for five years, until a dispute over his future led him to start his own practice.

What makes veterinary medicine so satisfying and exciting for Gene Solomon begins with the animals with whom he experiences "an immediate emotional entanglement," but also has to do with the city to which he is equally devoted. "Manhattan is the best place in the world to be a veterinarian. Think about how many people live here," Solomon says excitedly. "Think about how we live—crammed together in tiny apartments in high buildings."

Dogs and cats are much more intimate parts of residents' lives in New York than anywhere else. It is more of a personal relationship—a genuine friendship with all of the inherent demands and insecurities. "Think about the special needs of the Manhattan pet. You have to take the animal outside. There aren't any backyards, even in the richest households. So he's got to be walked regularly, and in the process, you interact with him. You feed him. You're with him most of the time."

Because of the intimacy experienced with a pet, an owner will more often notice—and become obsessed by—normal health problems. How quickly do people discover that their dog has diarrhea if they live in the country or suburbs? "One bout here, an owner is on the phone; it's a genuine emergency in a two-room apartment, and they want me to do something about it right now, on-the-spot."

New Yorkers are very demanding in everything they do, Solomon explains, and that extends to what they expect from their veterinarians. They want to push the envelope of life, death, and survival. "Money is no object. I have eight or nine patients in the office right now that are 'carte blanche'—anything that's necessary to keep them alive or to discover the reasons behind the animal's pain and sickness."

Veterinarians in Manhattan, and for the most part all across the United States, are a congenial lot. In contrast to medical conventions in which impeccably dressed doctors pose and preen at seminars and discussions and rush from meeting to meeting, briefcase in hand, veterinarians together are usually relaxed and jovial, in khakis and Levis, running shoes and hiking boots, joking and back-slapping. Parties go late into the night. To the observer at such conventions, the veterinary profession is also close-knit. But back at the office, a week later, those same warm and cuddly animal lovers become businesspeople in which the bottom line, caring for animals and their owners, is clouded by salaries, hospital overhead, the constant purchase of equipment, and the looming reality of a fluctuating profit-and-loss statement.

Veterinarians are not literally hostile or cutthroat to colleagues—far from it; rather, their attitudes as businesspeople are ambivalent. It is as if their colleagues either do not really exist, or, conversely (if their existence is hard to deny), it is meaningless; the veterinary world that matters begins and ends in their small, private hospital. Veterinary ambivalence toward one another hinges on the reality that the stakes are so low and simultaneously so high. Veterinarians simply do not have the capacity to make a lot of money. The umbrella provided by health insurance in the medical world is basically nonexistent. So every client and every procedure is guarded zealously. The typical veterinarian believes that referring an owner to a specialist or another veterinarian for any reason is tantamount to giving away income. "You won't get that client back," a Manhattan veterinarian told me, as he leafed through the Yellow Pages business directory to illustrate how his animal hospital, once alone in the neighborhood, was being encircled by competition. Veterinarians must present themselves as all-knowing patriarchs (and matriarchs); knowledge and trust are their most valuable commodities for sale.

Working swiftly, Solomon, a blue paper hat and mask concealing his head and face, quickly gowns, soaps, scrubs, and dries his hands, snaps on a pair of surgical gloves, arranges a set of blue towels around the surgical field, lifts a scalpel—and cuts. A couple of flicks of the wrist, and he's suddenly groping around, elbow deep inside the poodle's abdominal area, as if reaching for a glove or cap stuffed into a coat sleeve.

"This dog came in two days ago. Swallowed a sock." Solomon had waited to see if the dog passed the sock or parts of the sock in its stool before taking action. "But the dog was getting sick. He couldn't pee. His spleen was inflamed. An emergency exploration was required. 'Foreign bodies' often cause serious problems," Solomon said. It will take at least another half hour to locate and meticulously remove the remainder of the sock and sew the dog back up again. Foreign-body surgery, often time-consuming and challenging, is a routine part of domestic veterinary practice.

"Close your eyes and imagine," Solomon tells me, " 'foreign body' possibilities are limitless. Cassette tape, rubber balls, tennis balls, lingerie, jewelry, elastic strips, fan belts, and once, a set of eyeglasses—this from the littlest dog you've ever seen with the biggest mouth imaginable." And coins, pennies made before 1982, which were 97 percent copper, are less harmful than coins after that date because the composition changed; they became 97 percent zinc. And zinc destroys red blood cells, thus causing the animal to become extremely anemic, a life-threatening condition.

Cats are the most difficult foreign-body cases. Strings seem harmless, but Solomon was once confronted with a cat that was bleeding to death because a string had wrapped around the intestinal tract, shrunk, and sliced the bowel in half. Solomon removed thirty inches of bowel and saved the cat's life. During the Christmas holidays, tinsel is very popular for cats to swallow. "I actually met one of my fiancées through foreign-body surgery. Her dog swallowed a rubber toy, and she came to our hospital, panicked. I calmed her down."

Solomon, age thirty-nine, has never been married, but is no stranger to entanglements and engagements. Like medical doctors, police officers, and others involved in all-consuming professions, Solomon is obsessed by his work. "My mother said that from the time I was five years old, I was bringing animals home and trying to take care of them." He offers a flourishing gesture with a feces-caked clamp, forcing everyone in the room to flinch or duck their heads. "Today, I do house calls all over the world: Florida, California, Jamaica. Clients that I've met over the years, some of whom have moved away, would rather fly me down to wherever they are than get a new doctor. Some of the wealthiest people in the world. I mean, *in the world*," Solomon says. "I have a client who just left yesterday to go to Paris with her dog on the Concorde. The dog sits on the seat next to her, the two of them together."

A need to know often distinguishes the Manhattan resident from most other clients. When people ask, "What do you think caused my dog to get this condition?" the New York veterinarian is usually given permission to do diagnostic tests, skin scraping, blood tests, X rays, biopsies, tests that may be informative, but not cost-effective. "People in the suburbs say to their doctors, 'Look, what made my dog get sick?' And the veterinarian says, 'Well, if you want to find out, it will cost you $150.' And they say, 'That's too much. Fix the dog. I don't need to know why it happened.'

"But Manhattan has a great number of people without children, a great number of people who are by themselves. The animals become members of the family. As a result, you get two people who are living together; they have two incomes; they have no kids; they have no tuitions; they are consequently able to give the animal the kind of care that a typical suburban family, who can't afford to go the full nine yards, won't." On the Upper East Side, veterinarians will seldom euthanize animals because owners can't afford to care for them, a more common occurrence elsewhere.

As Gene Solomon continued his painstaking task of removing the swallowed sock, thread by thread and inch by inch, he explained that cats, from an anatomical and physiological point of view, were wholly unique. "One Tylenol in a cat is a good way to put them to sleep forever, whereas in a dog Tylenol is not as damaging." Cats lack the liver enzymes to metabolize Tylenol correctly. For those cats who do metabolize it, Tylenol becomes an oxidizing agent. "Their blood turns brown. Their membranes turn brown. A cat can die from just one Tylenol within twenty-four hours without treatment." Cats also hide disease better than dogs.

Concealing pain and sickness is part of the natural animal instinct to live life with bravado as a first line of defense against natural enemies. Animals are also unable to communicate physical deterioration. By the time such an easily treatable problem as glaucoma is diagnosed, for example, an animal may be blind in one eye. Dogs and cats cannot tell their owners that they have a headache or cannot see. Animals may experience pain and sickness in the same manner that people do, but they accept such discomfort and inconvenience as a way of life. In most veterinary emergency centers, trauma—auto accidents, dog fights, cats jumping out of high-rises—are most prevalent, as well as toxins, rat poison, and antifreeze being the most common.

Understanding the animal anatomy is perhaps the most awesome and ongoing task for a veterinarian—and a primary way in which to distinguish between the challenges and complications of human and animal medicine. The human is probably the most sophisticated animal, but humans are also miraculously and consistently similar despite differences in age, race, and nationality. Cats, dogs, and birds, for example, are entirely different, physiologically and anatomically. Each animal presents a unique anatomical challenge.

Some veterinarians, especially those in rural areas, will treat any species that cross the threshold of their office or hospital. Solomon and Schwartz have chosen to narrow the range of the species they are willing to treat to dogs and cats and other domestics to which clients in this prosperous neighborhood take a fancy. Although they are basically general practice, occasionally Schwartz will perform acupuncture, while Solomon is known for his work in oncology.

"Yesterday," said Solomon, "I put to sleep a patient who has been with me for three years. It was my hardest and most difficult case, ever. The owner, Pauline Wilson, was committed and obsessed. She was on the phone to me, literally, in the three years since we first met, at least once a day. No matter where I was in the world, she talked to me, sometimes half a dozen, sometimes a dozen times a day. Her cat had bone cancer of the jaw. I operated, removed the jaw. Cured the cancer. That was two years ago. But from that point onward, the animal had to be fed by hand. Pauline and her husband were willing to do this four times a day, day after day, for two years. And if that animal missed a meal or was off a little bit, they were on the phone, hysterical. This animal could not really walk around very well, but you see, the cat was happy. It watched television and looked out the window, and the family was comfortable with that."

"But *you* weren't comfortable," one of the veterinary technicians assisting with the surgery interjected.

"But it doesn't matter if I'm comfortable, subjectively speaking," says Solomon. "I only had to be comfortable objectively. Do you follow? 'Subjectively' means emotion . . . how I feel about it personally. Which has nothing to do with what is right or wrong. Objectively, I knew that animal was not suffering. Objectively, I knew that animal was not in pain, so I was fulfilling my responsibility as a veterinarian to the owner and the animal, and I could live very easily with that."

"How much money did Pauline invest over the three-year period in which you were treating the cat?" I asked.

"Enormous amounts," Solomon replied. "She could spend five hundred dollars a week in here. Easily. Listen," he shrugged and continued, "I have many clients like that. I am always honest with them. I'll say, 'To get your animal from here to there, say six months of life, will cost ten thousand dollars,' something like that. People will go for it. Money is not an issue in this practice.

Pauline loved her cat—lived for her cat; she refused to give up on her cat. Many people don't understand the deep level of emotion that the loss of an animal can cause on a human being, but after so many years of being together, losing a pet can be like losing a spouse or a child—or sometimes worse." Pauline Wilson invested more than fifty thousand dollars over a three-year period to keep her beloved "Baby Cat" alive.

Just then, as if on cue, a neatly groomed, nattily dressed man in his early forties pressed his nose against the window and asked Solomon through an abbreviated set of hand signals if he could enter. Solomon nodded and the man disappeared, then quickly reappeared, awkwardly arranging a blue mask and cap and easing himself into Solomon's surgical inner sanctum. "How are you doing today, Jason?" Although Solomon can be hard-edged, wisecracking, and cynical, his tone and manner visibly softened when Jason entered the room.

"I'm doing Okay, Gene," Jason replied. "Better than yesterday." Jason paused and swallowed. He lowered his head. Suddenly, without warning, he began to sob. "Gene," he choked, ". . . Beau. It's been a week and a day since he died."

Solomon continued to remove pieces of feces-caked sock from the dog's small intestine. "This has been a very hard time for you, Jason, but it's understandable not to be dealing so well. You and Beau were together eight years. If this was easy—for any of us—then we wouldn't have been so invested in our animals. The burden of our grief signifies the greatness of our loss."

Once again, Jason dabs his eyes and blows his nose. "I really am sorry," he says to no one in particular.

"There's nothing to be sorry about, Jason," Solomon assures him, as he neatly and nimbly completes the process of stitching his patient. In Manhattan, "cosmetics" are priority. Owners are very sensitive as to how much hair is shaved prior to the surgery, as well as to the extent and predominance of the scar after the surgery is completed. Finally feeling satisfied with his work, Solomon backs away from the table. He pulls off his gloves and tosses them into a nearby wastebasket, motioning to Jason to follow him. Fifteen minutes later, Jason appears once more. Again, he has been crying; his red face glistens with tears. But he is also calmer, and he is clutching a small corrugated cardboard box tightly to his chest as he leaves the hospital.

Later, Solomon is sitting in the cluttered office he shares with his partner, his hiking boots propped on his desk, while he wolfs down a roast beef sandwich and chugs a two-liter bottle of Pepsi. At first glance, Gene Solomon looks completely unlike any veterinarian one would imagine. He's young; his black hair is swept back in front; his teeth are widely spaced apart. He talks fast and walks fast; his style and mannerisms are much more reminiscent of a Manhattan attorney than a veterinarian. He is talking about Jason. "At first, he was kind of a distant friend I would see once in a while, socially, but we became much closer last year when I began giving his dog chemotherapy. Beau was a great dog and a brave dog. The morning of his death, he played for a few minutes in the park. It was a bittersweet ending."

That day, after Beau and Jason returned home from the park, Solomon canceled his late afternoon appointments and walked to Jason's apartment. In the living room, they talked quietly, Solomon all the while assuring Jason that he was doing the right thing, the only thing he could do for the dog and faithful friend whom he loved, considering the circumstances. Now Jason removed the bottle of champagne that had been chilling in the ice bucket on the coffee table, popped the cork, and poured two brimming glasses. They lifted their glasses slowly, and both men, owner and doctor, toasted their friend Beau in a very special and personal way. Then Gene quickly took the hypodermic needle that he had readied the moment he arrived and quickly and quietly injected Beau with sodium phenobarbital. Beau shuddered just once and settled for one last moment of togetherness into Jason's lap. He died quickly.

"Jason was here today to pick up Beau's ashes," Solomon tells me between bites of his sandwich and phone messages related by the office manager over the intercom. "He was feeling quite vulnerable. That's one reason he was so emotional in the operating room. This is the final part—and he feels foolish for wanting to keep the ashes with him at home. He told me: 'People will think it is weird.' "

"And what did you tell him?" I asked.

He shrugged. "There wasn't much to say," Solomon replied. He chewed thoughtfully, then leaned forward, wiping his hands nervously on his black Levis and smiling sheepishly. "Well, you saw where we went." He pointed out the door in the direction of the corridor in which he and Jason had disappeared. "There's a cabinet back there where I keep a few important personal possessions, and that's where I took him."

Solomon had opened the door of the cabinet for Jason, reached up to the top shelf and proceeded to pull out a leash and a collar and a jar of ashes from a dog he had euthanized. "This was my dog," he told Jason. "She died a little less than two years ago, but I keep these ashes close to where I spend most of my time. So, Jason, I guess I am just as weird as you."

# RESCUE FANTASY

The reception room in Solomon and Schwartz's Center for Veterinary Care at 236 East 75th Street is tastefully decorated, with framed photographs and watercolors of a variety of animals, including greyhounds and elephants. The dramatically curved reception desk is enhanced by a painting of a golden retriever on an adjacent wall. To one side of the desk is a large aquarium with tropical fish gurgling against a glass block wall. Behind the desk are rows of color-coded files. A long, green, L-shaped bench for clients is surrounded by a number of books concerning pets and animals and wildlife conservation.

Past the reception area, the bottom level of the building, which was in an earlier incarnation a bordello and is now owned jointly by Solomon and Schwartz, is roughly divided into three segments, beginning with a pet supply store, also part of the Solomon-Schwartz partnership. Both doctors are somewhat

reluctant to discuss such a commercial venture and rarely rec-
ommend Pet Necessities to their clients, although most of the
medications and specially prepared dietary foods and supple-
ments they suggest or prescribe are readily available next door.
Their reluctance stems from the notion, shared by most veterinarians, that seeming to be too commercial—selling leashes,
toys, and so on—diminishes prestige. But in reality, many veterinarians earn important income by selling products in tandem
with their own services.

Statistics show that offering pet products to clients is sound
business practice. According to a 1995 survey by the American
Pet Products Manufacturers Association, 63 percent of dog owners say they buy gifts for their pets, primarily at Christmastime;
45 percent of cat owners and 37 percent of bird owners say they
do the same. (Interestingly, in the same survey, more than 42
percent of cat owners and 25 percent of dog owners say that
their pets sleep in a person's bed at night.) In total, Americans
spend $20.3 billion annually on their pets, with about half that
amount going toward health care. The Humane Society esti-
mates that dog owners spend nearly $1,400 annually on their
pets, and cat owners about half that amount.

Behind Pet Necessities is a wing of empty rooms clients often
call "purgatory" because it is where owner and pet are escorted
if, for any reason, they are out of favor with the doctors or if bad
news must be communicated to an especially emotional owner.
Theoretically, the offices in this wing have been reserved for the
associate veterinarians Solomon and Schwartz periodically hire
and sometimes fire; it has been very difficult to find associates
willing to work as hard as they do, enduring the schedule and
the pressured demands of their clientele, even despite financial
incentives. Currently, the purgatorial wing is occupied by Amy
Attas, who will stop in with her technician/assistant and her
private driver a half-dozen times a day for supplies, to make

telephone calls, or to discuss a case she wants to refer. Recently, Solomon has been performing most of Attas's surgeries since her immobilization by a cat bite.

The hospital itself, located on the other side of purgatory, contains a kennel for overnight stays (the CVC has twenty employees), an isolation and X-ray area, an operating room, and four examination rooms, all clustered around a larger procedures room, where most of the daily treatment and animal-human or human-to-human interaction takes place, including the inevitable and ever-present dirt and mess.

On this particular day in the procedures room, weeks after Jason's outburst, Lisa, a tiny woman in her early twenties with brown hair, wearing blue scrubs, is sitting on a dry peninsula in the midst of a gigantic lake of urine, petting a small white hairy dog, a West Highland terrier called Annabelle, who is the reason Gene Solomon is dragging himself around this morning, unshaven, tired, and huffy.

Yesterday, after going through a tooth cleaning and examination and then taking a bath and sitting for a moment under the drier, Annabelle collapsed mysteriously, and for a while Solomon thought he had lost her. When she was revived, her eyes were very red and she seemed to be experiencing vision problems along with ecchymosis, a red blotch effect all over her body. Solomon doesn't know exactly what happened to Annabelle, although she is showing symptoms of heat prostration—and shock. Meanwhile, Norma, the chief technician, a former backup singer for the popular 1970s group Purple Mountain, is in the process of making fun of the name of the cat she's working on at this moment, Antigone. "My pets have normal names like Rick," she says.

Everyone at the CVC and seemingly most Manhattan veterinarians refer to pets as patients and owners as clients. The owners' last names are given to the pets' first names, and so there are a lot of funny names. As Cynthia and Diane the two receptionists move back and forth from the reception area, bringing patients for Schwartz, Solomon, and their corps to examine and treat, names are called off:

"Cubby Feldman!"

"Cock Duncan!"

"Frisco Farkas!"

Kala Silverstein is a pregnant Labrador retriever who's been defecating and vomiting in the house. Cynthia hands Solomon "a love letter from Mrs. Silverstein." He tears open the envelope and reads a vivid description of Kala's gastrointestinal difficulties, as seen through the dog's eyes.

A technician named Julio boosts Kala onto a stainless steel table and, pumping with a foot pedal, lifts her to waist-high position for examination. The table will also record Kala's weight, but she is frightened, squirming, and whimpering. Solomon immediately begins to address Kala as if she were a baby in a crib. "No one is going to hurt my little Kala, my honey girl," he says. "Kala is a breeder. She lived out in the country for her whole life until now. The Silversteins have to understand that she never had to live in a Manhattan apartment building or walk on the street with eight thousand beeping, honking, nasty cab drivers. She's having trouble adjusting."

Solomon's way with dogs is interesting and endearing. He likes to imitate or impersonate the dog by wrinkling up his nose and hanging his hands in front of his chest like paws as a way of greeting and of making friends, and then kiss it or pretend he kisses it by making kissing sounds with his lips. This approach seems to be acceptable enough to the animal, who will usually remain ambivalent, but very popular with the owners, who often expect—and need—to have their pets validated at every opportunity. Clients' self-images and emotional health are often intimately identified and integrated with their pets. This is not only true in Manhattan, but everywhere, city or country, and for all pets—horses, llamas, and scorpions included.

It is to Solomon's great credit that he approaches animals in the same endearing way when he is not being observed by clients. In his office or in the procedures room, he will repeat his little love dance and, if anything, become even more animated and uninhibited with animals away from the public's eye. "Dr. Solomon! Dr. Solomon!" Lisa's panicked voice suddenly echoes through the room, as she points down at Annabelle in her lap, who is suddenly twitching and trembling quite violently, as if someone is holding her up and shaking her silly.

Solomon passes Kala Silverstein back to Julio and observes Annabelle for a long instant, glancing at his watch. He then announces calmly, almost soothingly, to Lisa, "She's seizing. Nothing to worry about. It was only thirty seconds." He lifts Annabelle onto the table and begins to prepare an injection of medication, an anti-inflammatory; Annabelle continues to seize, her little body quaking rapidly. Valium will control seizures, but he doesn't want to "gork her up" unnecessarily, Solomon says. "It's very scary to see this little white furry dog of perhaps fifteen to twenty pounds, who is evidently weakened and in shock, suddenly start to shake. But it will be alright, not to worry." It is not clear if he is speaking to Lisa—or himself. "Seizures usually come in clusters. When you seize, the rapid fire of the neurons compound the action of the seizure."

Annabelle is now shaking so violently in Solomon's arms that she begins to squeal and yip in terror. Solomon injects another dosage of anti-inflammatory, but Annabelle's response is to shake and yip even more. Finally, about ten minutes later, Solomon decides to do what he initially resisted and "gork her up," or tranquilize her with Valium. He does so with a kiss and a soothing comment: "Your mother loves you," he croons.

Norma and Julio, the veterans, have been going about their

work on Frisco Farkas and Kala Silverstein in silence and without so much as a glance in Annabelle's direction. But when the
Valium takes effect and the crisis has clearly passed, everyone in
the treatment area gathers around Annabelle to make cooing
sounds and to pet her—gestures of reassurance to Annabelle and
to one another.

Solomon assigns Lisa the role of support for Annabelle.
"She'll be frightened when she wakes up, so I don't want you to
leave her alone."

This is very much a continuation of the theme I have observed in veterinary practices wherever I go, that the patient is
not abandoned just because the procedure has been completed
and the medical staff has other responsibilities. Solomon and
Schwartz are paying Lisa an hourly wage simply to comfort their
patient, a tiny and fragile animal, but certainly not any more
vulnerable and frightened than a human. Lisa actually crawls
into Annabelle's cage and cuddles up beside her, kissing and
petting and singing while sitting in a pool of urine. "I ruined
three scrubs today. Here goes four."

Throughout the afternoon, Lisa maintains her vigil, periodically rearranging the pad on which Annabelle sleeps, carefully
folding the blanket and talking to Annabelle as if she was a real
human being, as if Annabelle understood exactly what Lisa was
saying. Periodically, Solomon will look in on Annabelle and
make his kissing noises, while imitating the cute little tilt of her
tiny furry head. "Hi, Dr. Solomon," he coos in a childish voice.
"I'm feeling better now, thank you."

The staff at CVC and in most other veterinary milieus I have
entered into don't seem to communicate or relate to one another in any significant personal way, except for their shared
interest in animals—animals they're caring for at that particular
moment, animals that are in the hospital, animals they have
seen before and are wondering about, animals they own. And

when they do talk, they more than likely will be talking to the animal rather than to one another. Occasionally, Solomon will mention the Baltimore Orioles, in whom he has an impassioned interest. Schwartz, who is the administrator of their practice, will broach a business-related question. But basically, for everyone involved in treatment at the CVC, animals are the consuming force of their lives.

Near the end of that day, I was approached by Aldonna, the office manager, who was accompanied by a chic, red-haired woman, stylishly dressed in a rust-colored blazer, matching slacks, olive green turtleneck, and brown shoes. "You've been wanting to meet this lady," Aldonna says. "This is Pauline Wilson."

I could hardly believe it! Pauline Wilson, the real Pauline Wilson, the obsessed owner of the famous Baby Cat. The woman Solomon had been so upset about and had discussed with Jason. Solomon's most difficult and challenging patient. But Pauline Wilson bore no resemblance to the image that had formulated in my mind. Listening to Solomon discussing Pauline—a conversation that went on incessantly (there was no end to Pauline's legend and the legacy of her persistence, even though Baby Cat was dead)—I had been repeatedly reminded of James Herriot's nemesis (and friend), Mrs. Pumphrey, an elderly widow whose late husband, a local beer baron, had left her a large fortune with a beautiful house on the outskirts of town. She lived there with a large staff of servants, including a gardener and a chauffeur and her beloved Tricki Woo, a Pekingese terrier and, as Herriot says, "the apple of his mistress' eye."

When Herriot called on Mrs. Pumphrey, he was always welcomed with trays of cocktail biscuits and bottles of sherry, and gigantic packages of gourmet foods were sent to Herriot on holidays. And Mrs. Pumphrey always yelled to Tricki at the instant of his arrival, "Here's your Uncle Herriot!" Before examining

Tricki, Herriot was escorted into a large bathroom with a dressing table, toilet articles, and a bath towel for the ritual handwashing. When Tricki went on vacation to the shore, "Uncle Herriot" was sent boxes of oak-smoked kippers, and when the tomatoes ripened in Tricki's greenhouse, he was sent a pound or two of tomatoes every week, not to mention tins of tobacco and sometimes even a personally inscribed photograph of Tricki.

But Pauline Wilson was not the meek, dowdy Mrs. Pumphrey type. Rather, she was a sophisticated and articulate woman who began discussing the colors of my tie, the cut of my blazer. I asked her to lunch. We walked up the street to a local restaurant and talked for two hours. We met again a few weeks later and talked four hours more. She was obsessed with Baby Cat's death—and with her relationship with Gene Solomon. "A relationship with an animal is like having a terminal child," she told me, "because you know from the beginning that their life span is short. The reality of it is that you better enjoy every damn day you've got with them because your time together is so fleeting."

Remarkably, she found meaning in her two-year fifty-thousand-dollar struggle to keep Baby Cat alive. "Baby Cat kept surviving and responding to Gene's treatment because he wanted to stay around to make sure that my husband, Dick, and I stayed together. Because, you know, this kind of thing breaks marriages up. I have a couple of friends who lost children and it ended the marriages. Wonderful marriages. And the basis of it really is that both parties in their own grief cannot deal with one another. So the other one gets belligerent or resentful. And they drift. If Dick and I hadn't been able to work together on Baby Cat, all of our little squabbles about our businesses, plus locking heads on procedures relating to Baby Cat, might have ruined us. Baby Cat was witness to our many disputes. Baby Cat used to look at us both and shake his head, like, 'You two, when are you going to get your act together here?' I think he was testing us."

\* \* \*

When I arrived at the Center for Veterinary Care the following morning, Annabelle was lying in her cage in the procedures room just as I had last seen her. "How's Annabelle this morning?" I asked Norma, who was standing beside the cage.

Norma looked at me, woodenly. "Gone," she said.

"Gone? But isn't that Annabelle?" I nodded down at the cage.

"Yes," said Norma. "She's dead."

I couldn't believe it. I stooped down and began to pet her for lack of anything better to do.

"That's why Dr. Solomon is looking so sad and ragged this morning. He was up with Annabelle half the night."

Tomorrow Annabelle will be cremated and returned to Solomon in a special urn. Most people want their pets cremated, and they request that the ashes be returned. But only 25 percent of those owners who want the ashes actually claim them. "I have a whole room of urns with ashes," said Solomon. The urn with his dog Cathy's ashes remains in the cabinet in his examination room. "My patients like to know it's there."

Solomon walked into the procedures room, looking lost and distracted. He has a very heavy walk, so you always hear him coming. And he eats nervously through the day, muffins that his girlfriend has baked, candy; whatever people bring in, he eats. And he does it rather noisily, smacking his lips with each bite.

Solomon remained distracted through the morning until a clone of Annabelle suddenly arrived, named Austin. Solomon calls Austin "my remission dog. This is my second favorite Westie, actually my first favorite Westie now that Annabelle has died. I cured Austin of cancer. We gave her chemo and she lost all her hair."

"She was positively naked," Norma says.

"Now look at her coat," Solomon says, picking at the white curly fur and admiring how thick the coat has grown in.

The phone rings. It's Annabelle's owner calling Solomon to ask about the ashes. She wants to make sure that the ashes in the urn she receives will really be the ashes of Annabelle and not some other dog. This question has come up because of a scandal not long ago concerning one well-known pet cemetery that would cremate dogs but save money by avoiding the task of cataloging the urns.

Solomon assures the distressed woman that the company he is dealing with is legitimate, and then ambles into the kennel area and grasps a gigantic tabby cat by the scruff of its neck. This is Mylo, whom Solomon has owned for five years. Mylo seems to have the run of the place, but he is so big and so assertive that few other creatures would have the nerve to get in his way. Solomon sits down on the floor, cross-legged, his stethoscope dangling from his neck, playing with Mylo and glancing at the newspaper. As he plays he begins to wheeze and clear his throat loudly. His voice becomes husky and hoarse. Then he begins to cough. Solomon is allergic to cats.

At this point, another Westie comes in for a manicure and grooming. "Dudley," says Solomon, "is a be-careful kind of dog because he will bite your face off. Actually, he bit one of the children in his family. His owners came to me for my opinion about what Dudley's outlook for life should be. I told them that a dog that bites people, unprovoked, is not a pet. I recommended training to make sure that Dudley would be controllable or to find Dudley another home without kids. Or to put Dudley to sleep. That was five years ago. I don't think they did any of the things I suggested."

"But he hasn't hurt anyone since?"

"Not that I know of," Solomon says.

Solomon owns two dogs. Biscuit, a three-year-old golden retriever and V. C., a three-legged mutt. V. C. was seven weeks old when she came into his office. One of his clients had been in a taxi when the driver revealed that three days before he had rescued a dog hit by a car, which he saw cowering in the street, its leg shattered. The driver took the dog to a nearby veterinarian who wanted too much money to euthanize it—and so the driver took it home, where it was lying on the floor on a blanket. Solomon's client was so upset at the driver's story that she forced him to drive home to get the dog, and the client took the dog to Solomon, who promised the taxi driver to put the dog to sleep. But the more he looked at the shattered leg, the more he felt he wanted to try to save it. He labored over this leg in surgery for a long time—unsuccessfully. When he amputated the leg, he decided to keep the dog. "No way I could put that dog to sleep. I named him V. C. for 'vet care,' and also," he said, " 'very cute.' " V. C. lived at the Center for Veterinary Care until Cathy, Solomon's original golden retriever, died. Then Solomon took V. C. home to be with his new golden retriever, Biscuit. "V. C. has become Biscuit's surrogate mother," Solomon said.

Later he is teary-eyed when asked about the death of Cathy, who had cancer. "We do a lot of cancer treatment in New York. Perhaps more than in most places," says Solomon. "Can't exactly tell you why. I can tell you that the golden retriever is one of the most popular dogs and the most susceptible to cancer because of the inbreeding that occurs because of the demand. German shepherds, too, and boxers are also very popular and susceptible to cancer. Jason's golden was eight when he died. I kept him going an extra two years."

Cathy, however, died prematurely on his operating table during exploratory surgery. "I felt her heart and suddenly I knew—I said, 'Something is not right.' His anesthesia machine had malfunctioned—the only time that such a malfunction, which might occasionally happen, had led to the death of an animal.

"For a while, I couldn't work. I couldn't stop crying. I couldn't face any other dog." Schwartz, who had been on vacation for the week, was called in to take over. "What bothered me more than anything was that I never said good-bye. Suddenly she was dead and I never said good-bye. I couldn't eat or drink or sleep. I did nothing but sob at home for three days. I lost my mother not long ago, the most important person in my life. And I was less upset because I was more prepared. I was not prepared to lose Cathy."

Pauline Wilson once told me that the loss of Cathy had been the key to her close relationship with Solomon. "There was a wavelength we shared, and every once in a while, when I really thought I was going to fall apart, Gene would be able to say, in one or two sentences, something that would put all of the doubt or fear in perspective. Gene understood my love for Baby Cat, which is in sharp contrast to a number of my closest friends. During my ordeal, many friends ignored my crisis with Baby Cat. Never Gene."

As much as she respects and appreciates Solomon, they were often at odds; their personalities would clash. "He's impatient. He's argumentative. He does not respond to authority, and he does not like accountability. I called him up and said, 'Gene, I'm coming to have a meeting with you. I want you to block out the time.' Paid $175. And we went at it. My accusation was that Gene was being perfunctory in his treatment of Baby Cat because he never petted him. I said, 'I think you like dogs better than cats.' But an interesting thing would happen after all of our many fights. After we screamed and yelled there would be this opening up—a breakthrough. He would come into the room where I would be cuddled with Baby Cat, sit down on the floor, and we'd have this good conversation. We would confide some aspect of our personalities that would give reason for our behavior. Women have such communications as a matter of course, but men require a special situation, a crisis, especially Gene."

Pauline's assessment of Solomon is accurate, according to Solomon himself, with whom I shared Pauline's comments— with permission. "I don't like to hear this stuff, but I can't deny the truth in them."

Paul Schwartz shrugged when he read Pauline's observations. "That's my partner," he concluded. "But I still love him."

# OFFICE HOURS

A s the day passes and the flow of clients with their pets and problems increases, Solomon seems to warm up and relax. He consults with a Filipino woman in a white uniform who brings in another Westie, a popular breed on Manhattan's Upper East Side, with stomach problems. Later, he says, "We have a big housekeeper practice here. I've had clients for years, and I've never met them, personally. If I was having dinner with them, I wouldn't know who they were, until I heard their voices. These are people I talk with on the phone quite a bit, but see only their housekeepers face-to-face. We get letters, we get faxes, we get notes from owners, telling us what to do with their pets."

He shows me a letter written on personal stationery of one of his best clients, a well-known writer and a former TV producer, who has written him a note, ostensibly from her dog, explaining what needs to be done, as if the dog is talking, and not the owner. In fact, she signs the dog's name.

Solomon's next client is a fashionable woman in a red satin coat, black turtleneck jersey, black stockings, black suede shoes, very tight cheeks (obviously having had one or more face-lifts), and dyed blond hair. She tells Solomon that she has three questions and promptly begins: "Is it normal for dogs to lick furniture?"

Solomon answers that it is and that it is a natural response of any curious dog, especially when they are alone.

"And when I put a goodie on my knee" (the woman takes her finely manicured fingertip and places it on her knee) "is it normal for my dog to nudge it with her nose rather than eat it?"

"Yes," says Solomon, "to see if it is alive."

"And why," says the woman, "does my dog scratch at my rug?"

"Like he's trying to dig a hole to China?" Solomon jokes.

"Exactly," she says.

"Actually he's looking to build a home. That's all it is. It's all normal animal behavior."

The woman nods. "My real concern is her bad breath. Is there mouthwash I can buy for dogs?"

Next, Mary Tyler Moore's dogs are brought in by her secretary, a middle-aged male who tells Solomon about his employer's TV pilot, her feature films, and the editing of her autobiography. Mary Tyler Moore has two dogs, but this dog, a Petit Bichon Griffith, essentially a basset dog with short legs, whose name is Dudley, is having bowel movements eight times a day.

Solomon says: "Does anybody give him snacks or treats?"

"No one but Mary," the secretary says, as if her contributions to the dog's gastrointestinal problems cannot count.

In addition to Mary Tyler Moore, Solomon's famous clients

have included Joan Rivers, Henry Kissinger, and Si Newhouse, publisher of *The New Yorker*.

Later, Mrs. Lynn Goldstein wants to know if Skippy can have her body rolfed (a vigorous technique of muscle manipulation) to calm her down and make her feel better.

"No," says Solomon, "since her bones are brittle from thirteen years of prednisone, body rolfing is not a good idea."

A few minutes after saying good-bye to the Goldsteins, Julio bursts into the room with a squirming, screeching bundle, wrapped in a blanket. This is Missy the Cat who is such a wild, ill-mannered holy terror that Schwartz and Solomon charge double for nail-cutting. "It is like casualty insurance," Solomon says. Missy the Cat is the meanest and most dangerous cat of all of their feline patients. "You never know what that cat is going to do; she's a walking time bomb." The second-to-the-most-terrible is named Miss Marvel Miller, who, Solomon learns, happens to be in the waiting room at this very moment.

"Missy the Cat and Miss Marvel Miller," Solomon shakes his head. "This is shaping up to be a very difficult day."

It's interesting to watch Solomon and Schwartz try to make the transition from paying attention to animals to paying attention to children. A friend carrying an infant in a car seat stops to say hello. "This is my son," the father announced proudly. Schwartz glances at the baby as if it is a book on a shelf. "Very nice," he says, nodding cursorily and walking away.

Solomon is friendlier, but his greeting is noticeably less enthusiastic than the greeting he gives to dogs or cats. Norma says: "I never cared much for children, so it didn't seem a smart idea to have any." She has three dogs and two cats.

After going through his getting-acquainted kissing dance with a pudgy brown springer spaniel suffering from chronic diarrhea, Gene Solomon says to the heavyset, well-dressed woman, accompanied by her teenage daughter, "Tell me what you feed her."

The woman gulps and lowers her head.

"Yes, tell him, Mother," the daughter says.

"Chicken."

"Chicken," Solomon nods calmly and writes something into the dog's chart. "Anything else?"

Once again, the woman gulps, as if she's been caught in an act that she had been trying to conceal, which, of course, is absolutely true. "Fruit," she says.

"Fruit?"

"Yes, raisins, bananas . . ."

"And kiwi," her daughter adds.

Solomon nods again, writes in the chart and carefully eyeballs the patient. The woman's daughter is now smiling widely, on the verge of laughter.

"Any normal food?" Solomon asks. He is straightforward and matter-of-fact. He does not make any attempt to call attention to this odd dietary regimen. "I mean, normal dog food?" he corrected himself.

Again the woman swallows. "Well . . . bagels," she says.

"Well," says Solomon calmly, "bagels are better than fruit and chicken, but if you intend to continue to feed her chicken, then take the skin off—and eliminate the dark meat."

"But she likes dark meat."

Solomon shrugs. "White meat is best for dogs, in the chicken category."

"She really prefers dark meat," the woman repeats.

"Well," says Solomon, "if she's that picky . . ."

"Okay, okay," says the woman, "I guess I can do that."

Now the daughter bursts out laughing. Solomon, however, remains calm and deadpan and maintains a professional distance, while continuing to pet and kiss the little brown dog with the floppy ears. The mother, who has been growing increasingly uncomfortable, is now blushing; she has moved far back into the corner of the examination room. She sinks down to the ground, covering her face with her hands. "What's wrong with you, Mother?" her daughter asks.

"Oh, I feel so stupid."

Above her head on the wall is a fancy framed photograph with Solomon and Cathy. There's also a small bulletin board with dozens of photos of pets, pets and their owners, litters of dogs, paintings and drawings of pets, and a framed poem entitled "The Precious Gifts He Gives, A Tribute to Dr. Gene Solomon."

Solomon calls for a technician to retrieve the dog so that a few tests can be conducted, and then addresses the woman and her daughter about the many years of intestinal disease that their dog has suffered and how a consistent proper diet would help stabilize the dog's health—and increase its longevity. They spend a good deal of time discussing animals and nutrition, trading questions, answers, and ideas until the woman interrupts by asking, "What about grapes?"

"Well," says Solomon, continuing to be both sincere and matter-of-fact without indicating signs of annoyance, "a springer spaniel's ideal diet will probably not include grapes."

Now the woman addresses her daughter: "I really have to get Joel to stop feeding him French food on Saturday afternoon."

Solomon interjects: "I actually have less of a problem with croissants than I do fried chicken."

The woman looks up, hopefully. "So croissants are good then?"

"I wouldn't go that far," Solomon says.

As we leave the examination room and walk down the hall toward his office, Solomon's face reddens and he shakes his head with disgust. "How many times has she been here?" he says, flipping the pages of the chart. "Twenty times? Thirty times? And what's the first question I asked her on her first visit?" He flips back to the beginning of the chart. "Diet. 'What do you feed your dog?' We go through this every time at anywhere from $75 to $250 a visit. And she will not listen. I would pay the $75 or $250 if she would only listen—just once. That woman is a very well-known, highly accomplished psychotherapist in this community. That's the kind of clients we have here. They know exactly what they want to do about their pets and they know exactly what they want from me. Their message is consistent: 'I don't care what it costs.' That's what she first said, right? I want you to fix up my dog good as new . . . so that I can kill him with kiwi and croissants."

Schwartz and Solomon share one tiny office, cluttered with boxes, files, journals, shopping bags, briefcases, pieces of equipment, envelopes, paper cups, empty Pepsi cans, and a large bottle of Rogaine, which is for Solomon. "That woman who fed her dog chicken and croissants," he tells me as we settle into our chairs, "has been a client for six or seven years. She listens to everything I say. Sometimes commits it to memory and often quotes me, word for word, when she returns for the next visit. It's a shame," he says, "for this woman loves her dog." He pauses and expels a deep breath. "For the most part," he says, "owner compliance is a norm in Manhattan, and on the other hand, when dogs get sick, very often it's because of owner noncompliance.

"Pauline Wilson was a wonderful owner. She took such a careful detailed history, and so meticulously described the symptoms on yellow legal pads and in her careful tiny script so that I could understand and define Baby Cat's problem. She wrote

down every drink of water. Every feeding. Every bowel movement that she observed. She writes like this," Solomon imitated
a minuscule, birdlike scrawl in the air with his fingers. "Pauline
spent a chunk of her life in room three."

Room three is the visiting room. "We offer clients the opportunity to spend time with their pets who have to stay with us
overnight—or for many nights. Our clients can come in whenever they choose; they are allowed free access to room three, just
as Pauline had for seven weeks, twelve hours a day during Baby
Cat's chemotherapy. We encourage visitation. Human contact
makes an animal feel better, reduces the stress of being in a
foreign place. We have had vigils here, all night, all week, over
dogs and cats. We have had candlelight ceremonies on behalf of
the dog's health and recovery. If animals are cerebrally intact,
they will usually respond to human kindness and attention. In
fact, an animal, even in a coma, will sense their owner's pres-
ence and respond positively. In turn," he says, "the owner often
needs psychological support the veterinarian can provide."

We talk briefly about the healing power of animals—in many
different venues—until Paul Schwartz comes into the room, sits
down in a chair, and picks up the tail end of our conversation.
"Mind if I tell him the 'Steven' story?"

Solomon shakes his head—he doesn't care. Schwartz, a short,
slender CPA lookalike in need of a haircut, leans forward and
begins. He has a very pronounced New York accent and talks, as
does Solomon, with constant and elaborate hand motions. "Picture in your mind," Schwartz says, "the prototypical 1968
hippie-type."

Solomon interrupts. "Ponytail. Old, rotten, scuffed up, worn-
down boots. Filthy Levi's. This guy, first time I saw him, is laying
down on the bench in our reception area, his feet propped up on
one of the tables, unshaven, looking a mess. And I wanted to
throw him out. I thought he was a street person."

"Meanwhile," says Schwartz, "back in the examination area, I'm examining his dog, with his wife. The dog was suffering from liver disease, from liver dysfunction. It was a very serious situation."

"And I was ready to throw him out," Solomon repeated.

"Yes, that's what my partner here wanted to do." Schwartz nodded. "Until I told him who this 'street person' actually was."

"Wasn't I surprised!" said Solomon.

"Did you ever hear of Bruce Springsteen? And the E Street Band?" Schwartz asked. "This was Steven Van Zandt, the lead guitarist and songwriter slouching on that bench with his eyes closed, not because he was a slob but, on the contrary, because he was so terribly distressed. Steven was overwhelmingly committed to his dog. During the most delicate part of the treatment, at least three weeks in the hospital, Steven would come here at four P.M. every afternoon and stay in room three with his dog until two A.M., sometimes longer. He said to me more than once 'Dr. Schwartz, this dog cannot die. I will not allow you to allow my dog to die. You must keep him alive.'

" 'Steven,' I always said to him, 'I'm doing the best I can.'

"One time, he pulled me into room three. And he started to cry. 'Doc,' he said. 'This dog is my life. This dog keeps me alive. He cannot die.'

"Another time, he says, 'Doc, I'm doing a new album now. This album is very important to me. But I'm getting desperate. I can't work. I can't think without my dog. You've got to get him home for me.' Well, it actually took three weeks, but we cured him, and we sent the dog home. Steven was very happy.

"One of the reasons our practice is successful," Schwartz says, "or one of the reasons people like coming here, is because it is so private. Owners can allow themselves to become upset—safely, unembarrassed. This place is an emotional outlet and as private and sacred as a psychiatrist's couch.

"Let me ask you," Schwartz says, propping his feet up on the desk. He's wearing pointed-toe cowboy boots and black Levi's today. "What's the worst thing that can happen to a human being? I'll tell you what the worst thing is. It's rejection. Rejection is the worst thing that can happen to a human being."

Now he leans forward and lowers his voice. "And animals never reject their owners. That's one of the beauties of owning animals. Dogs and cats can be trusted with the intimate feelings of their masters. So a great bond begins to develop between an animal and its owner. Animals are always so supportive. Especially when the animal and the owner have a lot of contact. And when their animals' lives are endangered, in any way, shape, or form the owners often, no matter how sophisticated and successful they are, cannot endure the strain and the fear of loss. And they break down and often confess all manner of things that are embarrassing and demeaning. You hear stories and confessions that come out of a person's mouth, and you want to say, 'I'm not your shrink. Go see your shrink. I'm your dog's doctor, for God's sake!'"

"It is very strange," says Solomon, "when people tell you about their innermost fears and how somehow those stories and anxieties are directly entangled with their pets."

"I've talked to psychiatrists about what people have told me in my office," Schwartz continues. "Psychiatrists are astounded. 'You mean they come in here and they spill their guts out?' Yes, I say. Sometimes, they've never seen me before. They will tell you everything that is terrible about their lives on the very first visit. They bare their souls. This is such a funny place," says Schwartz, "with so many strange questions."

Schwartz's approach to animals is quite different than Solomon's. He doesn't play with the dogs or cats. He's cursory, at best; he deals with the animal in a businesslike manner, as he does with the owner. He just launches into the examination straight away and talks to the client, nonstop. There's a sign under his name on the wall on a shelf where telephone messages are put; it says, "Won't he ever stop talking?"

"Remember the truck driver?" Solomon asks.

"The truck driver!" Schwartz replies. "Who could ever forget the truck driver? He was at least six feet four inches tall. I do not exaggerate. He weighed 250 pounds, I swear. When I told him his puppy had liver disease, he broke down and began weeping. He collapsed on my shoulders. He was so big and so heavy that my knees buckled, and I fell to the ground; he toppled over top of me, bawling like a baby. It was gruesome."

Pauline Wilson's tantrums will also always be remembered—by Schwartz, Solomon, and Pauline herself, especially the day she learned that Baby Cat had cancer. "I was stunned. I fell on the floor by the fish tank in the reception room at CVC. I couldn't believe it. Dick, my husband, tried to pick me up, but I pushed away, got up and walked outside. The car was parked across the street and I sat in it for a while. All I can remember is that I was so confused, so frustrated, I was beating on the steering wheel with my fists."

Schwartz and Solomon understand that the Pauline Wilsons of the world are an intricate part of private veterinary practice. "We see six to seven thousand animals," said Solomon. "That's our patient base in any given year. About five hundred of those animals come here on a regular basis, that is, weekly or every few weeks for baths, allergy shots, or normal examinations—whether they need them or not. Sometimes owners have a need for their animals to be examined, and the people themselves need to be listened to. And we will often do that listening."

Now Solomon takes a telephone call from a client with a twenty-two-year-old cat with one eye who wants to know what it's going to take to make her pet feel—and see—better. Solomon refers her to a veterinary ophthalmologist then hangs up the phone. "That's actually the oldest cat I ever operated on," said Solomon. "Twenty-two years old."

Schwartz says: "I examined a cat who was thirty-one. When the owner told me her cat was thirty-one, I said 'No way.' But then she said, 'His name is Groovy.' So then I believed her."

"Behind everyone who comes in here—all my owners—is a story," Solomon tells me. "One of the reasons I left the Animal Medical Center after my internship is because I was just a tool for caring for pets. There was no relationship between me and an owner. It was a hospital atmosphere. There was no story. The story is why I am in business—people and their animals and their lives together—and why we run the kind of practice we do."

Solomon's father died when his mother was five months pregnant with him. She supported the family as a government employee but was constantly in debt. He has two older siblings. He discusses his reasons for attempting to save and then deciding to keep V. C. as a pet—and how that decision connects to his philosophy of veterinary medicine and his background. "When I was a kid, my first dog was hit by a car. I was in school at the time. My mother took my dog to a veterinarian, who didn't think he could save the leg nor did he think the dog could live for too long with its handicap." He leaned forward and raised his voice. "Therefore, the vet assumed that the dog would not want to have only three legs and therefore the vet put this dog to sleep. I had nothing to say about it. I never had a chance. I never had a choice. My dog did not live because someone did not want to go to any trouble to give me a choice. That doesn't sit well with me. It never has. It never will.

"In veterinary medicine, there's often no right or wrong decision. What counts is what's appropriate for the owner. I give them all the options. I give my clients the choice that I never got when I was a kid with that little dog. They decide what they want to do; no one decides for them. Then I ask them if they want my opinion, and if they do, I will give it to them. Now, certainly, if the treatment is cruel and inhumane, I will not do it. Nor, in fact, will I put an animal to sleep if it is not a medical euthanasia.

"Or if it is a medical problem and someone comes to me to put the animal to sleep and I see that the problem can be treated, I will treat the animal. I will treat the animal at no charge before I would put it to sleep, unnecessarily. Animals have as much right to the best care and treatment as humans do. God created us equally."

# A Way of Life

The first veterinarians have been traced as far back as ancient Babylonia, two thousand years before the birth of Christ. Records document a fee given to a man for treating a cow; the man was subsequently penalized when the animal died—perhaps the first recorded case of malpractice. Hippocrates, who was so influential in the development of human medicine, was similarly so in the development of veterinary medicine in about 350 BC. And in India, a century later, King Asoka ordered the construction of the world's first veterinary hospital—a revolutionary vision unequaled in the Western world until 1762 in France at Lyon, where a center was established to search for ways to control cattle plague, which was decimating most of the livestock herds in Europe. By the end of that century, there were twenty veterinary facilities in a dozen European countries.

The first veterinary college in the United States, the Veterinary College of Philadelphia, now part of the University of Pennsylvania, was established in 1852. Prior to World War II, the peak of veterinary medical education, sixty-eight veterinary colleges were active; today only twenty-seven remain, twenty-five of which are land-grant institutions, supported primarily by state and federal agricultural subsidies. Tufts University in Boston and the University of Pennsylvania are the only two private veterinary institutions, perhaps the two finest veterinary colleges for their overall educational impact, but often treated in the veterinary world with a certain amused and jealous disdain.

Penn graduate veterinarians are known as "Pennwees," allegedly such overbearing know-it-alls that they frequently begin conversations with other veterinarians, no matter what the context, by saying: "At Penn, we . . ." Penn graduate veterinarians are always recognizable because all other veterinary schools bestow a DVM (Doctor of Veterinary Medicine) degree, while Penn provides an VMD (Veterinary Medical Doctor) degree. "Do you know what VMD stands for?" veterinarians are constantly joking whenever a Penn graduate is about. "Very Much in Debt." As private institutions, Penn and Tufts are by far the most expensive of all veterinary schools, nationwide.

Originally established to offer technological support and training to offspring of farmers and ranchers in the rural United States, colleges of veterinary medicine have been traditionally difficult for city-bred students to enter—especially out-of-state residents. In many areas of the country it has been more difficult to gain entry into veterinary school than medical school. Wendy Freeman worked as a technician for two veterinarians while in high school. "I applied five times to veterinary school. I applied as a junior in college, senior in college. I applied the first and second year of my master's program in exercise physiology, then the year after that before being accepted."

Freeman's grades, education, and experience were acceptable, but not her sex. Norma Harlan, a veterinary inspector for the U.S. Department of Agriculture (USDA) applied three times to Ohio State Veterinary School before being accepted in the late 1970s. In the large building in which her anatomy lab was located, there was only one ladies' room. Today, more women are becoming veterinarians because of the elimination of discriminatory practices and because the profession often permits a flexibility that allows for children and family. Many women are working part-time for established practices or joining large superstore operations such as PetSmart.

The basic fact that some women are content to labor as part-time professionals and work for far less money is thought by many male veterinarians as undermining to the profession. As in any small business, establishing a practice requires, at least in the beginning, anywhere from a sixty- to an eighty-hour workweek, plus a substantial financial outlay. Settling for an hourly wage as a subservient and uninvolved employee plays into the hands of big business, which is out to consume the veterinary practitioner, some people think. PetSmart and operations like it are, if nothing else, symbolically threatening in a world in which 80 percent of all professionals are involved in a practice of two or fewer people. "After PetSmart and the other superstores become ingrained," a veterinarian told me, "there won't be many of us independents left for you to interview."

But new ideas and modern technology have threatened veterinary life for as long as anyone can remember. Long before James Herriot began to practice, the average veterinarian devoted most time and effort to treating horses used for farmwork, freight transport, and basic transportation—a gradually diminishing necessity after the introduction of the automobile. After World War II, medications were developed that, when fed to growing chickens, controlled coccidiosis. This breakthrough enabled farmers to expand to gigantic, highly concentrated sites for poultry operations with perhaps as many as a million birds on a single farm. Subsequently, the poultry industry learned to deal with nutrition, housing, disease control, and genetics. Veterinarians, wedded to the concept of responding to calls on small or medium-sized family farms and treating individual sick animals, were unable to fit into such production-line operations. Similarly, other sectors of the livestock industry have intensified production practices, while learning to rely less on veterinarians.

Not that veterinarians have been totally stripped of their role as overseers of the public health. Veterinarians in regulatory medicine, primarily employed by the USDA, will protect the public from diseased livestock and unsafe meat, poultry, and dairy products. Veterinarians in public health capacities investigate disease outbreaks, such as rabies or ringworm, evaluate the safety of food-processing plants and restaurants, and help determine the efficacy of drugs used on animals and humans. There are thousands of veterinarians in military service, including many like those featured in Richard Preston's best-selling nonfiction book *The Hot Zone*, which demonstrated the potential human devastation of uncontrolled animal-originated viruses. In private industry, veterinarians may specialize in pharmacology, microbiology, bacteriology, pathology, toxicology—and even sales and marketing.

A profession of relatively young people (the mean age is thirty-nine), there are positions available for veterinarians in zoos, circuses, animal theme parks such as Sea World, as well as in space medicine, fur ranches, and in education. Before personal taxes, a veterinarian's net income is approximately $70,000 for an average fifty-two-hour workweek, although first-year income directly out of veterinary school can be as low as $15,000. Average starting salary for a graduate DVM is $27,000 annually compared to $42,000 for an MD.

Despite modest rewards (considering a decade-long education), veterinarians in the United States have a better life than anywhere else in the world, according to Van Roy Meit, a visiting veterinarian from Belgium whom I met at New Bolton Center, Penn's large animal hospital. Veterinary education in Belgium is inferior compared to schooling in the United States, Meit said, and the political system around which education and civil service employment is anchored is backward and corrupt. "We buy the same books in Belgium, but the equipment is missing. It is so frustrating. In the U.S. when an animal needs help at ten P.M., someone will respond. But in Belgium at five o'clock, it is quit."

We are sitting in the cafeteria at New Bolton. Meit says that in her country many sick animals die unnecessarily because of an unwieldy and unenlightened bureaucracy. While a student, Meit read a book entitled *Equine Clinical Neo-Natology* by Wendy Vaala, VMD, which is what brought her to New Bolton for further study the year after graduation. "My boss doesn't know that New Bolton exists."

Meit's friend, Subine, is sitting at our table. Subine is an aviator veterinarian, meaning that she is hired on a freelance basis to care for horses being transported intercontinentally. On any one flight, as many as twenty-one horses can be transported, along with 220 passengers. Horses are placed in containers of three horse stalls situated on a palette. Seven palettes will fit in the tail of an aircraft. Usually, one veterinarian is assigned to each container, so there may be as many as seven veterinarians on any given flight. When arriving in New York, the horses are inspected at the "Vetport," a facility adjacent to Kennedy International Airport.

Subine, slender and dark-complected, says: "Most people don't become veterinarians; they are born with a calling to animals. Animals are better 'people'—than real people. Animals are open in everything they do. They kick you, but you can see them kick. They are not doing it behind your back. Working with animals is less a profession and more a way of life. Human doctors care more about treating disease, whereas veterinarians care about patients. You have a client. You go to a farm. You have a cup of coffee. You treat the animal. You become part of family life. When you are partying with veterinarians, there are more animals than kids."

"Do you have children?" I ask a New Bolton nurse who is listening to our conversation.

"Yes, I have kids," she laughs—"four-legged ones. Five cats, two horses, and three dogs. That's all I can handle."

There are few opportunities available as an aviator veterinarian or a racetrack or vetport veterinarian, but these positions reflect the surprising scope and potential of the veterinary life. According to the American Veterinary Medical Association (AVMA), approximately 80 percent of the sixty thousand veterinarians in the United States today are in private practice, more than half of whom engage in small animal practice, meaning pet animals, primarily dogs and cats. There are five thousand boarded specialists in nineteen AVMA recognized specialty boards and colleges, including pathology, oncology, and behavioral medicine, the newest approved specialty, in which antidepressive medications such as Prozac can be prescribed for dogs and cats.

Right now the field is in deep turmoil, with veterinarians attempting to shape the future of the profession and decide who and what they want to be. An important distinction between veterinarians and human doctors is that veterinarians' patients can be many different species, whereas doctors deal only with the human species. In many respects, that's what veterinarians are trying to decide as they contemplate their future—whether they should become a practice of specialties. The current licensing exam asks questions about all species, and when you are licensed, those who pass are licensed as veterinarians and not as specialists.

Throughout the history of their profession, veterinarians have prided themselves in being doctors for all seasons, all maladies, all species and breeds. But the concept of boarded specialties in human medicine has made significant inroads in the veterinary profession. It is ironic but typical that the leaders in veterinary medicine seem more inclined toward specialization just at the point at which human doctors, who have embraced specialties vociferously for the past thirty years, are now rejecting them.

At the time James Herriot began practicing in England prior to World War II, there were no specialties whatsoever in veterinary medicine and animal medications were made from scratch in makeshift laboratories. Before going out on the road to call on clients, veterinarians loaded their cars with carefully compounded potions and powders, which Herriot admits, in retrospect, were largely useless. Veterinarians were careful physicians, but relied on many drugs for a placebo effect on worried and impatient animal owners.

Herriot writes about one popular product, UCM (Universal Cattle Medicine), which he describes, tongue in cheek, as the last line of defense in the battle with animal disease. A rich, red fluid with the strong aroma of camphor ammonia that always impressed farmers, and packed in tall, shapely bottles with labels that declared in big black type its efficaciousness, UCM was said to cure, among other diseases, "the scowls, milk fever, pneumonia, felon and bloat." The label also advertised a slogan: "Never fails to give relief." Herriot read the label so often that he half believed it, he said, even though everyone, especially veterinarians, considered UCM useless.

If veterinary medicine is a profession for those men and women who dream of an idyllic lifestyle with animals as its centerpiece, it is also a profession with disappointments, with some specialties like exotic or wildlife areas nearly impossible to penetrate. I was visiting with a group of veterinarians who had attended a lecture at a zoo one day, walking with them and listening to their conversations as they toured the complex. One man with a couple of cameras was in his early or mid-thirties, slight, clean-shaven, wearing running shoes and casual clothes. Because of the cameras, I assumed that he worked for the zoo or for the public relations agency representing the zoo and that they were doing some sort of publicity story. When we began talking, I learned that he was a veterinarian in practice in a private twenty-four-hour animal emergency center in the suburbs. I asked if he enjoyed the veterinary life. First he smiled, but then an incredibly sad look burst upon his face. For a moment, I thought that he was going to cry, he seemed so distressed. "I'm sorry but this is not a good day to ask me," he said.

We were silent for a while as we walked through the complex, but I pursued the issue. Was the profession making him unhappy? Or the place where he worked, which employed eleven veterinarians? "I'm becoming overwhelmed with the stress of the life I have to lead, and the money that I make, which certainly doesn't equal the hours I put in," he said. "And people don't regard me with much importance; even my family would rather I be a medical doctor, not an animal doctor. The place where I work is very busy. Because it's an emergency center, people don't have to make appointments. They come in helter-skelter, whenever they want, and they're scared and unhappy, and they don't talk in a nice way, and they don't like to wait, and they're worried about their animals and how much the treatment is going to cost. And so it's not very pleasant."

"Did you always want to be a veterinarian?" I asked.

He had been interested in snakes and alligators and before attending veterinary school at Ohio State, had earned a master's degree in herpetology. The only real possibility of working with snakes was to work in a zoo, and those jobs were so rare that they weren't even worth pursuing. "Being in vet school was a lifelong dream. People said I wouldn't get into school, it was so competitive. And people said I wouldn't make it through, it was so difficult. But I succeeded; it was very exciting.

"The admissions people in vet schools choose very carefully. They want candidates interested in two hundred different kinds of species—intellectual and scientific heavyweights—renaissance men. They want people with open minds, who will be challenged by different kinds of adventures. And so they recruit and accept those people, and then they work you so hard and angle you in such a manner that before you know it, all the reasons that they accepted you—great versatility, flexibility, intelligence, athletic accomplishments—are squelched. When you get out of school, you find out that all of the things that you dreamed about doing as a veterinarian are practically impossible." After a while, he said, "I'll tell you, if I had it to do all over again, I wouldn't be a veterinarian."

In a similar story, Brad Bentz, a recent New Bolton graduate, owes $110,000 in loans, while his brother, who started medical school at the same time, owes $90,000. Bentz says he has a twenty-year payment book, "like a mortgage on a house." The average educational debt of graduating veterinarians, not counting undergraduate loans, according to the AVMA, is $41,000. Bentz worked in a private equine practice directly out of school, but unlike James Herriot, found it frustrating; the financial and emotional rewards were small. Horse ownership is a status symbol in certain parts of the country, conceived and defended as a constitutional right by some people as vociferously as others protect their right to keep guns, except that horses cost a lot more money to feed and care for than do gun oil and ammunition.

"A lot of horses are owned by the wrong people," he said. "People with mobile homes. People with duct-taped windows and doors that are bailing-wired together. People with eight kids. They call you, and they want you to do many procedures on their horses, and you know in your heart that everything you are doing for these horses is taking bread off the table for their children. I constantly felt like a crook."

Bentz was also mistreated, along with the animals. "People made the horses live in the freezing cold, which is where I was expected to treat them. They gave you freezing cold water to clean up the wounds. No heat. Knee-deep in mud. And as much as I wanted to question them, I had to play their ball game. In private practice, you've got to make people believe that you are very pleased to be where you are and doing what you are doing—or they will call someone else. Or they will ridicule you and deny that your diagnosis is accurate."

Obstetrician-gynecologist Patricia Sertich is sensitive about the skewed image of the veterinarian in today's world, explaining that the practice has changed significantly since the era about which Herriot wrote. "People don't realize we have every bit as much training as human doctors; people will differentiate between veterinarians and 'real doctors,' as if we're impostors. I feel very respected by my clients, but other professionals often regard me as someone who plays with animals. We don't play with animals. We take care of them; we do the same diagnostic tests as all doctors do on humans. We don't get much respect. MDs talk down to me."

Though the first two years of veterinary school and medical

school are essentially the same, Susan Cohen, a social worker at the Animal Medical Center in Manhattan, the largest small-animal hospital in the world, who counsels and teaches veterinary students, observes that a number of the interns complain that people ask them, "Do you have to go to school for this? Are you a real doctor? You're not a real doctor, you're a veterinarian." Cohen says, "I once heard a mother say, 'My son is graduating from vet school and my other son is a doctor.'"

Of the veterinarians with whom I have been in contact, many are surprised at the direction their lives have taken since graduating veterinary school; their particular role or place in the veterinary life is quite different from the world and the lifestyle they had initially imagined. Arthur Bramson, for example, who thought he would be treating dogs, cats, and parakeets in a suburban domestic animal practice, today supervises five veterinarians, five veterinary technicians, and approximately sixty support personnel at the University of Pittsburgh Medical Center, which maintains a population of twenty-five thousand animals for research.

Not long ago, dogs, particularly beagles, were the research animal of choice for surgical experiments, but not anymore. "Pigs are a lot cheaper," Bramson says. "And the vast preponderance of animals for experimental laboratory work are rats and mice. There are rabbits, chinchillas, ferrets, gerbils, guinea pigs, hamsters, some sheep. I don't know if you're aware, but there are catalogs of rodents to purchase for medical research—probably five hundred different inbred mutant stocks from which to choose." The University of Pittsburgh also owns about thirty-five baboons to use in experiments for xenografts—animal-to-human organ transplants.

One of the first veterinarians I interviewed, Jonathan Allan, works at the Southwest Foundation for Biomedical Research, the facility that supplies baboons and chimpanzees for research and transplantation to hospitals across the United States. Allan, who had dreamed of being a wildlife veterinarian since childhood, moved to Michigan and worked as a bartender while studying virology in graduate school and establishing residency in the state. Massachusetts, where he grew up, did not have a state-subsidized school of veterinary medicine, and the tuition at Tufts was too high for his family to afford. Eventually, he earned his DVM at the University of Michigan, "but after finally achieving my dream and going through veterinary school, I knew in my heart I could never practice—at least in the traditional sense." Allan discovered that virological research, especially the seamless connection between the simian immunodeficiency virus (SIV) and HIV in man, interested him much more.

There are currently 2,700 olive, red, yellow, chacma, and hamadryas baboons at Southwest, where Allan conducts his research, with 200 more born every year, and 225 chimpanzees. The campus, located on seventy-five acres of Texas prairie dotted with scrub brush and black mesquite trees two miles from Sea World, is an eclectic collection of rambling single-story asymmetrical buildings housing offices, laboratories, and banks of animal cages. The buildings twist and turn around a series of elaborate and awkwardly contrived cyclone fence corrals, filled with swinging, chattering, jumping, screeching nonhuman primates.

Allan refers to himself as a virologist rather than a veterinarian and completely isolates himself from the animals he infects. Yet, eye level on Allan's bulletin board are four photographs of Jack, a black mixed-breed dog who died at age fourteen. "I got him at the pound when he was eight weeks old. He went everywhere with me. But I don't have a dog anymore since Jack died and I started working here," Allan said.

Administrators at Southwest share Allan's ambivalence to animals, creating an atmosphere for the animals that is oddly reflective of the human experience. Chimps involved in AIDS research (chimps do not die from AIDS, but must remain in lifetime quarantine) live in "condos" or "duplexes" in a cinderblock development called Infectious Village. Each unit has a palm tree, a patio, four-seasons temperature control, indoor plumbing, and a color TV to watch. Their favorite programs are *Mr. Rogers* and *Geraldo*.

Although focused on animals, Allan and other veterinary specialists labor for the benefit of mankind. On a baseline level, the world depends on animals to provide a variety of necessities. Livestock and fish are what the majority of Americans eat; conversely, poor nutrition is the world's leading cause of death, meaning that the value of food-animal veterinarians is more precious than ever. Horses, dogs, and cats contribute to our psychological well-being. Zoo animals and wild animals add to the quality of our lives, while a great variety of animals contribute to scientific research. A cure for AIDS or cancer, as with most every medical breakthrough, will most certainly have begun with laboratory work on animals. Such indispensable research is ongoing at every major human and veterinary medical center in the world.

# VHUP

He was bearded, tall and slender, towering over the people with whom he stopped to chat. His dark brown hair, parted in the middle and streaked with gray, fell haphazardly over his shoulders. This man was interesting to see, but what attracted me more than his physical appearance was the way he moved, or glided, as if his height and his striking, mystical appearance connected him to some other world. I followed him into his office and sat down in a chair across from his desk. The man said that his name was Mark Haskins, and the poster behind his head contained the following message: DISEASES ARE NOT CONQUERED BY PEOPLE ALONE.

The disease that Mark Haskins is attempting to conquer at the Veterinary Hospital of the University of Pennsylvania (VHUP) in western Philadelphia is mucopolysaccharidosis (MPS I), a genetic lysosomal storage disorder that causes significant physical handicaps as well as serious and irreversible mental retardation. The most well-known form of this category of diseases (lysosomal storage disorders) is Tay-Sachs disease. Other well-known variations include Hunter's syndrome and Gaucher's (pronounced gow-shays) disease. Several lysosomal storage disorders affect children who are Jewish, primarily the Ashkenazi of light-skinned, European lineage.

Lifting a long graceful arm and pointing at another poster behind my head, Haskins said: "The Siamese cat on that poster behind you illustrates the effects of MPS. Instead of having the nice pointed features of the Siamese, her face is flattened, her ears are small, and she's in a hunched up position because her spine is fused. She has hip subluxations, corneal clouding, a deformed chest and trachea, and enlarged liver. All are features you see in children with these same diseases."

Many children with MPS progress normally until they're two or three years old. They will start to develop language and toileting skills, and then they begin to lose those skills, become hyperactive, and much less interactive. Their IQs may be as high as seventy; they have a shortened life expectancy. Most will die before they reach their twentieth birthday. The first MPS animal was discovered twenty years ago at VHUP—the Siamese cat, on which Haskins wrote his PhD thesis. Siamese cats with MPS have subsequently been discovered throughout the United States and in Europe, and the first dog diagnosed with MPS was found in California. "We're trying to understand the pathogenesis or progression of the disease from beginning to end."

As an example of the progress that has been achieved—and the remaining problems—in one type of MPS, Gaucher's disease, Haskins explains that scientists have discovered that replacing a missing enzyme in people can stop the proliferation of the disease in the body immediately. But treating a child with this enzyme, manufactured by recombinant DNA technology, costs between $150,000 and $300,000 annually. Moreover, there are additional concerns, such as the advisability of giving intravenous drugs to people for the rest of their lives; if you stop for any reason, the disease comes back.

Another moral issue is the use of animals in medical research. One of the strengths of using animals is that certain controls can be established and tests conducted with a minimum of complications. Inbred mice, for example, are identical genetically, except for the mutation—a fact that can significantly enhance the learning curve. But the knowledge gained from mice may not be applicable to human beings, which is why the larger animal model is often used. Most of Haskins's work is supported by the National Institutes of Health (NIH) and the MPS Society, composed primarily of parents who recognize that the prognosis for severely affected MPS children is hopeless at present. But most of those children have siblings, many of whom are carriers, and whose decisions to have families will be significantly influenced by the development of treatment.

The NIH funding has little to do with animals, obviously, but veterinarians are more likely to be funded if their work benefits people; animals are, at best, secondary in research priority for most funding agents. This is not to say that there aren't veterinarians whose research concerns animal-oriented problems exclusively, but more often than not practicality dictates a dual objective.

The University of Pennsylvania has long set the standard for veterinary research in the United States, attracting more funding from the NIH than any other veterinary institution. VHUP is rooted in the university medical complex in Philadelphia, established more than a century ago by a group of physicians who believed that a world-class medical institution must be supported by an academic veterinary community in an atmosphere in which constant collaboration can occur.

Not too many years ago, horses, swine, cattle, and a myriad of other livestock and exotic animals were literally boarded and treated at VHUP directly adjacent to the legendary CHOP (Children's Hospital of Pennsylvania) and the medical school. Today, and ever since New Bolton Center was established, many of the classrooms and administrative offices are located in the bricked courtyard intake compound, where horses and livestock once lived. Not only was the veterinary complex inspired by doctors, but the first two deans of the school of veterinary medicine were MDs.

Haskins entered his profession "through a whole series of strange happenstances. My sister is seven years older than I am. She desperately wanted to be a veterinarian. But in the 1950s, there were few women in the profession. When she went to our local vet and announced her career choice, he said, 'Women don't belong in the profession.' And so she believed him—and became a nurse. Years later, when people began to ask me what it was I wanted to do when I grew up, I had no clue. So I said what my older sister said. I want to be a veterinarian. And that's exactly what happened."

After graduation, he hopped a freighter to Hong Kong, Manila, and Singapore, hitchhiked through Malaysia into Thailand and eventually Australia, before returning to Philadelphia to investigate the possibility of a master's degree in biomedical engineering. A series of chance encounters led to a job at VHUP and a somewhat providential meeting with a dwarfed Siamese cat named Suzie Reeves, who had MPS—the first to be discovered in an animal. "I wrote my dissertation, started to publish papers, and I've been doing it for twenty years."

Had he ever considered moving in a slightly different direction to obtain an MD? Despite his resemblance to a higher authority, Haskins replied in a most un-Christ-like manner: "I don't like sick people. My sister eventually ended up in an emergency room as a nurse. And I saw enough of what she had to endure to realize that it wasn't what I was interested in—not for a moment." But as Haskins and all other veterinarians have learned, emergency and intensive care medicine in a large veterinary hospital is as challenging, quirky, and heart-wrenching as in any high-acuity hospital for humans.

When I walk into the intensive care unit at VHUP, a crowd of doctors, nurses, residents, interns, and students are watching, flustered, as a large white cat, sprawled on the stainless steel examination table, connected to lines and probes, is quite possibly dying in front of their eyes.

The cat had come into the hospital with an arrhythmia and had suddenly arrested. The ICU staff had restored the heartbeat, lost it, restored it again, lost it, brought her back once more. Now she is being connected to a ventilator to keep her alive.

Joan Hendricks, a slender, soft-spoken veterinarian with short, graying hair, who is supervising the ICU today, and Meg Sleeper, the twenty-four-year-old resident in cardiology who was examining the cat when the arrest occurred, are discussing what to do—and what not to do—next.

"The ventilator is very uncomfortable," Hendricks says. "And all these strangers in white coats are poking her with needles and instruments. We don't know what she's feeling or thinking, but if she has any concept of reality, she must be scared to death." The situation is especially frustrating because they are working in the dark, keeping the kitty alive without any real insight into her underlying problem.

Hendricks asks Meg Sleeper if the owners have been given a financial update. Following standard procedure, Sleeper had initially estimated that ICU treatment would cost five hundred dollars, but the estimate has since been upgraded to a thousand dollars. The owners have communicated their desire to not spare expense. Sleeper is wearing a blue neckerchief around her hair, a yellow polo shirt, and dock-siders. She says to Hendricks: "This cat is so young and vital. I feel so sad in cases like these."

"You think it would help if the owners see her?" Hendricks asks Sleeper. Hendricks loves animals, but feels a strong obligation to help owners confront reality. A visit to the ICU, seeing their animal so encumbered with probes and lines, might help overcome the "She was okay last week" syndrome, enabling them to consider what is often referred to in veterinary circles as "that beautiful option of euthanasia." Sleeper moves to the desk in the corner and picks up a phone. There are twelve cages and two ventilators squeezed into this small windowless room made of cinder block, painted white, with a scattering of animals resting on mattresses, sheets, and pillows. A couch for cuddling, when a nurse, doctor, or owner wants to comfort an animal, is also provided.

The white cat is an unusual patient for the ICU because it was transferred from the cardiology department. The cat's cardiac arrest occurred during a routine examination. Most ICU patients originate in the emergency room. On a busy day, the ICU at VHUP might confront four new problem cases of varying origins: an animal with a ruptured abdominal abscess, a dying diabetic cat, a dog with a brain tumor, another with a raging fever, at least one traffic accident victim, and always a few animals, undiagnosed, which necessitates simultaneously "keeping the animal alive, and also solving the diagnostic puzzle," which is what is happening with the little white kitty this evening.

Meanwhile, Reid, a slight, neatly dressed young resident wearing a button-down-collared shirt, a stylish print tie, and a wrinkled white lab coat, enters the room. Visibly shaken, he approaches Hendricks quickly: "He's here," he says.

Last week, Reid had euthanized an eighteen-year-old golden retriever dying of cancer. The upset owner had understood the necessity of ending his old friend's life. He gave his permission to have the dog put to sleep, and after it occurred, had hugged Reid and thanked him for his compassion. During the following week, however, the man thought he saw his old dog hanging out in front of his house, but every time he opened his door, the dog disappeared. He began telephoning Reid to ask for further explanations about why his dog had really been euthanized—and if the dog had been euthanized, how these visits could thus be possible. Feeling pressured, Reid had reluctantly invited the man to the hospital for a brief consultation. Hendricks does not endorse Reid's generosity of time and spirit; she feels that the man sounds unstable, but has reluctantly agreed to attend the meeting. Reid has also asked VHUP social worker Kathleen Dunn for backup support.

Dunn, a psychiatric social worker who has been counseling pet owners at VHUP for more than a decade, donates her office for the meeting—a small, cluttered cube with three chairs, a coat rack, and a desk. I am happy to remain on the periphery with Dunn, who has previously offered to meet with the owner. He is a tall, bearded, and hulking man, about forty years of age, ominous in his anxiety.

Dunn and I position ourselves in the waiting area adjacent to the emergency room, directly across from her office. As we talk, we can observe the traffic moving in and out. I spent a great deal of time in emergency rooms in hospitals for my previous books, and I marvel at the similarity of the milieu. There aren't any ambulances moving in and out of the emergency room, but the basic scene is as frantic and bizarre as in any human hospital. People are double-parking their cars, looking concerned, waiting nervously for news from doctors; stretchers are being rolled in and out by harried men and women in blue scrubs and surgical gowns. People from all different walks of life have suddenly and rudely been thrown together sharing a silent and stoic aura of dread and fear.

Kathleen Dunn had been called from home the night of the euthanization to meet with this man, but when she arrived, Reid seemed to have the situation under control. That evening, after Reid and the man hugged and said good-bye, Dunn watched the man linger in the waiting area, muttering to himself and crying. She waited until he left the building and disappeared down the street.

The stages of mourning and grieving a pet owner suffers through is analogous to the process described by death-and-dying expert Elisabeth Kübler-Ross: From anger, either at the veterinarian who couldn't save their very ill animal, or at themselves for not finding a way to have prevented the animal's demise—to denial. Owners will often imagine that they see or hear their diseased animals, suddenly and mysteriously returned to life.

Dunn leads a biweekly support group for people who have lost pets. At a recent meeting, a woman cried so hard for her dead cat that she burst a blood vessel in her lung and had to be hospitalized. This cat had sustained her when her husband died, and had accompanied her on a trip to Paris; they had cruised side-by-side down the Seine. Very often, Dunn hears stories about human losses; the loss of a pet stirs memories of the loss of a human being in someone's life, a process she calls "linkage." A woman once came into the emergency room with a golden retriever who had nearly strangled itself with a rope to which it had been tied in the backyard. She was hysterical. Dunn, on twenty-four-hour call, was paged, and after a long conversation, learned that the woman's son had committed suicide by strangling himself.

Animals with cancer can stir up especially bad memories among owners who have suffered through the death of a loved one with cancer. Dunn has heard from colleagues at other institutions of five cases in which owners have committed suicide over the loss of their animals. Some owners of perfectly healthy pets will visit with Dunn on a periodic basis just to prepare themselves for the eventual loss of their animal. One lady threatened to divorce her husband because he wasn't mourning the loss of their cat as deeply as she thought he should.

There are people who are much too attached to their animals. One woman whose dog died in the VHUP emergency room suddenly decided to sit with the remains of her pet—after the autopsy had been performed. Veterinary pathologists are not as carefully cosmetic as are human doctors, but this women was determined to have a proper good-bye. The woman was given a room for privacy, where she sat for hours embracing her dog's entrails, which were floating in preservation solution in a plastic bag. The disposition of the dead body of the pet can also become complicated. Dunn is currently counseling a healthy forty-year-old businesswoman, who is arranging with her attorney for the ashes of her dead dog to be buried with her when she dies. Others want their pets buried in a place in the backyard where it liked to sit in the sun or play ball. Some people consider having the animal stuffed by a taxidermist.

How ashes are actually returned to owners is often critical. The hospital recently affiliated with a crematorium that packs ashes in a satin-lined cedar box with a purple ribbon. Previously, ashes were returned in plastic bags or cardboard boxes; Dunn has received numerous phone calls from people who got their pet's ashes back that way and want to exchange them for the cedar box option. Some people have asked that ashes be shipped to them Federal Express because they cannot bear to return to the site of their animal's death. Dunn also arranges religious consults: Priests and rabbis have visited the ICU to bless the dying or departed pet or conduct a ceremony.

The routine emergency room scenario at VHUP will not end in death. Average visits are usually serious, but not often fatal, concerning the swallowing of foreign bodies like superballs, strings, and coins. Sick-animal behavior problems are always worrisome. "If you can get a muzzle on the dog and get the dog away from the owner, there isn't much of a problem," a doctor told me. There are also a few tricks. "You take a leash and you run it through the crack where the hinges attach to the door. The dog's head is maneuvered into the corner so that the veterinarian can safely approach from behind. Cats are less predictable because they can bite and claw. Dogs have claws but they're not as sharp. Cats will rake you. They really dig in."

What works inordinately well in controlling cats is a fishnet. "Drop a net over the head; the claws get caught up in the mesh. And then inject the cat with sedative to proceed with the examination. Animals, like people, are not rational when they are in pain or very sick. They can bite themselves or fight themselves to death." Another problem in an animal emergency room is what is referred to as a "dump." People run in, drop the pet in the emergency room waiting area, and run out. You never see them again.

After about a half hour, Reid and Hendricks emerge from Dunn's office, say good-bye to the man, and quickly disappear down the hall. But instead of leaving, the man stops to linger with the owner of a golden retriever, who is at VHUP for a minor procedure, retelling his story from beginning to end. This time, however, he is blaming his local veterinarian for not referring the dog more promptly to VHUP. Hendricks tells me later that what this man wants more than anything is someone to blame. "But there is really nobody to blame. The dog was eighteen years old and it was time for the dog to die."

When we return to the ICU, Meg Sleeper is about to escort the owners of the dying cat into the unit. These people are very young and handsome, seemingly well-to-do, and in their early thirties. At first sight, the woman bursts into tears, kneels down, and attempts to talk to her cat. The man bends over his wife, looking concerned. After about five minutes, she jumps up, throws herself into her husband's arms, then wrenches herself away and runs out of the room, Meg Sleeper and the husband following.

"The owners want to wait a couple of more hours," Meg Sleeper reports back later. "The husband says that his wife needs more time to face the fact that they will not be taking their kitty home."

Now the doctors, nurses, students, and technicians have momentarily run out of things to do; they all stand around and talk. It is Friday evening, seven o'clock; a new shift has come on, but these people can't seem to go home. They discuss the possible causes of the arrhythmia, the difficulty of sinking an arterial line into a small cat, the frustration of doing all that they're doing for the little white kitty, knowing that they're really doing nothing for the sake of the cat—that is to say, nothing to deal with the problem that brought the cat to the ICU in the first place, but only maintaining the status quo, which is really being done as a service to the owners—and certainly not the animal who long ago disengaged with reality and awareness.

Meanwhile, Reid, who has served an internship at Texas A&M and is now in a three-year ICU residency, has left the building and headed home, but the bearded owner to whom he had said good-bye was waiting for him at the hospital entrance. But this time he was not abusive or untoward; in fact, he was overly solicitous, couldn't stop thanking Reid for all the good work he had done. "Is there anything I can do to repay you?"

"But it wasn't really me," Reid replies, "it was everybody in the ICU."

"But I need to do something. I haven't done enough to thank you."

"Send a basket of fruit to the ICU staff."

"No, that's not really enough. I owe you more."

"Well, then," said Reid, "send two baskets of fruit."

The white cat died an hour after Reid left the hospital, but the fruit never arrived.

I rendezvous at eight o'clock the following morning in the ICU with Joan Hendricks, where she is waiting with a can of Pepsi and her five-month-old bulldog puppy, Grumble.

Although Grumble lives with her at home, Hendricks, known in veterinary circles as the "bulldog lady," considers Grumble a colleague because they are both working toward the same goal— curing a potentially lethal disease that afflicts 5 percent of all animals and perhaps even a larger percentage of human beings: sleep apnea. Essentially, this describes a condition in which bull-dogs and humans stop breathing when they go to sleep, although they may not be aware of it. "Sometimes they do not breathe for more than half of the time they are asleep, and they will snore very loudly and wake themselves up and not know why." A portion of these people develop heart disease. "Sleep apnea is clearly a significant risk factor for being dead." All bulldogs de-velop sleep apnea, which makes for a very short life span (about five years), but they are also the perfect breed to use to study the problem and seek answers leading to a cure.

Hendricks suspects that sleep apnea has something to do with the shape of a bulldog's face, which forces them to work harder to breathe. Many people suffering from sleep apnea have round, flat faces and short bulldog-type necks. A surgical technique that basically consists of trimming tissue in the back of the throat has been moderately effective in extending life for both humans and bulldogs, but a cure is not possible until physicians know a lot more about the cause of the disease. Hendricks's colleagues at HUP (the hospital of the University of Pennsylvania) ask her the questions about sleep apnea to which they most need answers. "Maybe I can figure it out more quickly in my dogs than they can in people."

At New Bolton and VHUP, personal pets like Grumble are everywhere—and not usually for research purposes. Last night after Hendricks went home, I sat in the emergency room watching the patients coming and going, as well as the doctors, nurses, and residents. Most staff members had at least one animal. One doctor had thirteen dogs, large and small, on different variations of leashes, harnesses, and connections to other dogs.

"Where do you put these pets?" I asked Hendricks.

"Everywhere! Trish, a nurse, has two dogs in empty ICU cages. Grumble goes in my office. This is very much against the rules, and it's something we plan to address someday soon." While talking, she is examining an Emergency Service transfer sheet—a basic form filled out for each animal transferred from emergency room to the ICU, noting date, name of the clinician, and an estimate for how much treatment might cost, eight to fifteen hundred dollars in this case, with a five hundred dollar deposit. An emergency-room intern has summarized the case history:

"Dog came home, 10:19 P.M., having escaped. Was coughing blood and there was blood on hallway floor. Owner took to LV.M.D. [local veterinarian] and he thought that the dog was pale. And took rads of thorax. LV.M.D. found blood coming from mouth and nose and coughing continued and continued. Into Penn."

Hendricks proceeds to the X-ray screen to examine the film. The stomach is full of air, which could have been the result of a sloppy X ray by the local vet. There's fluid around the heart, which is probably blood. Hendricks is not only a researcher and an ICU specialist, but also an administrator in the veterinary school and opinionated about the importance of specialization and certification in certain veterinary areas—and the need to reshape basic veterinary education. In veterinary medicine, it is legal and common that after four years of training, a graduating student may receive a license and treat any animal—from a macaw to a moose. The graduating veterinarian can choose to be a surgeon, internist, pediatrician. But Hendricks feels that this is too much to ask from any human being: to know everything and to do everything right.

Should we be wary about our kitty or dog being cared for by someone just out of school?

"Yeah," she answered. "Absolutely. For anything that might be considered not routine, I would take my animal to a specialist."

Realizing the limits of their training, an increasing number of veterinarians are extending their education a year for a voluntary internship. If a particular specialty appeals to them, they may continue for anywhere from three to five years to become board-certified. The concept of specialized training and board certification is not easily accepted by older veterinarians whose entire philosophy and orientation has been rooted in independence and self-sufficiency. "These guys often think, 'If I can't solve the problem, nobody can.'"

After thoroughly examining the X ray on the screen, Hendricks speculates that the sick dog might have swallowed rat poison, which causes a great deal of internal bleeding. She and

Reid decide to do a clotting profile to assess the ability of the animal's blood to coagulate properly. Meanwhile, the dog's heart seems to be beating much too rapidly. Hendricks would like to use drugs to lower the heart rate, but is hesitant because, conceivably, with an elevated heart rate and internal bleeding, certain medications could cause an arrest. She decides to try to lower the heart rate with Lidocaine, and to consult with the cardiologist on call. The dog is a lurcher, similar in appearance to a greyhound or a whippet. A nurse says: "Some breeds that come into the hospital actually do not exist." She laughs, and then tells me about the "miniature chow" who was transferred into the ICU last week. "That's what the owner called the dog, although it was actually a pomeranian."

Two technicians arrive to fetch the lurcher for an X ray. "Until we know what's wrong, we're going to treat her with vitamin K, which is what you would do if rat poison was the problem," Reid tells me.

The cardiologist, a dark-complected muscular guy in his early thirties who arrives to examine the lurcher, looks at the monitor and says: "The dog is sick. Its heart doesn't like it." In other words, the heart is responding in protest. This commonsense, down-to-earth diagnosis is exactly true and reflects the extent of their knowledge at the moment. He watches for a while longer, and then says, "I'm now going to tell you what you already know. You have to identify and treat the underlying problem to understand what's happening with the heart." He is kneeling down, holding a stethoscope to the dog's heart, concentrating. At one point, a set of make-believe drumsticks appear in his hands, and he starts to tap out the heartbeat on the ICU floor. After a while, he gets carried away and begins to sing the distinctive beat aloud. (He reminds me of a young Mel Torme scat-singing.)

Hendricks asks if I want to feel the heart. I kneel down, place my hand gently on the dog's chest, and listen to the music in the stethoscope. The dog is very warm. The heartbeat is rapid, then slow, rapid, then slow. *Thump, thump, thump, thilly-ump-thump, thump, thump, thump.*

"Ain't that the coolest jazz?" the cardiologist asks. "I sure do love that beat."

The blood work has now returned from the pathology lab, but the results are perplexing. "Inconsistent with the rat poison theory," Hendricks says. "This is a case for a problem-oriented medicine man."

"Well," said Reid, "suddenly, this becomes a very interesting case."

As Reid and Hendricks begin to discuss their remaining diagnostic options, the nurses begin to plan their Christmas party for patients and owners who survived the VHUP ICU. Not every single patient who has passed through the unit will be invited, but dogs or cats who have remained there an inordinately long time, or who were really nice, or who had achieved some significant medical milestone, such as "most organs removed," "most blood products used," or otherwise established their reputation as "the couch potato dog," "the social butterfly dog," and so on.

They expect fifty animals and maybe as many as two hundred owners; last year, there were no fights between dogs, cats—or owners. The hospital pays to have the affair catered, just like a bar mitzvah. The nurses make invitations, bandannas, and special-award trophies. In the scrapbook of photos from previous Christmas parties, many of the dogs and cats are dressed up like Santa Claus or Santa's helpers. Everybody—animal and owner—has a good time. The nurses say that they do it in order to maintain some sort of contact with the patients, since the ICU is such an isolating experience. The clinicians may continue contact to communicate with owners and animals, but not usually the nurses. This year, they have invited Mayor Rendell's dog, Miss Woofy, as a surprise guest. Miss Woofy has accepted, but the mayor has not.

Meanwhile, Joan Hendricks can't understand what has gone wrong with their rat poison diagnosis on the lurcher. No other diagnosis computes, so she phones the lab to confirm the fact that the blood tests last night and coagulation test this morning have been taken from the right animal. After about ten minutes the lab phones back—to report a foul-up. The right dog—the lurcher—was tested, but the results had been abnormal. Curiously, instead of reporting the results, the laboratory technician had assumed that she had received the wrong sample. Now the mystery is solved, so treatment can proceed. The lurcher will be back at home with its owners the following morning.

# "Lady Comes into My Office"

Joan Hendricks's assessment of the general practitioner's limited capabilities is not disputed by Michael Obenski, a "kitty vet" who runs a cats-only hospital in Allentown, Pennsylvania. Obenski, a graduate of Penn, considers himself a member of the vast silent majority of veterinarians across the United States.

Obenski values what he calls the "sophisticated stuff" that VHUP can do, "but there's fifty thousand veterinarians in this country who are on the front lines where the real day-to-day work is being accomplished." Obenski, who is short and trim, with graying hair and glasses and who uses the words "peachy" and "spiffy" in most any descriptive framework, refers to his place of business, an old home that he has redesigned into a modern hospital for cats only, as "a tiny, yokel, small-time hospital" and himself as "a small-town yokel representing the 'silent majority' of veterinarians; I work from a Norman Rockwell painting."

He also works as a columnist for *D.V.M. News Magazine*, the only independent voice in the veterinary community. In a competition hatched by Obenski and *D.V.M.*, veterinarians from across the country were invited to write stories they most like to tell about their profession. Obenski received 327 entries representing a variety of interesting experiences, although Obenski also discovered the similarity of veterinary life—and the subjects veterinarians thought to be funny.

"There were at least fifteen stories in which the veterinarian diagnoses a dog as having trouble with the anal sacs," he said. "Owners become furious: 'How dare you imply my dog would have anal sex!' " In another set of stories, a dog's belly blows up and he starts passing stools all over the house. The stools grow bigger and bigger—right in front of the owner's eyes. This is because the dog has gotten into a container of bread dough that had not risen. "Veterinarians laugh at anything that is messy," Obenski said. "There were many essays in which the veterinarian lanced an abscess or lifted a cow's tail—and everybody in the room gets sprayed with an obnoxious substance. Veterinarians think that stuff is a riot."

Client ingratitude and/or obliviousness were also popular. A story of a farmer making an emergency phone call to a veterinarian about a cow with a prolapsed uterus, for instance. The veterinarian and his assistant rush out to the farm and spend hours freezing in the barn performing surgery. The farmer is nowhere to be found. Their job done, they go home. But when the farmer returns, he calls the veterinarian's office. "Tell the vet not to come. I just checked the cow and the uterus is back in."

Dead dog stories were abundant. "Clients show up at your office with their beloved dog—dead for two weeks. Some of them are so dead they smell." There are also clients who arrive for scheduled veterinary appointments with a stuffed animal or an alarm clock. "Sometimes people aren't right. You have to take care of them."

"Lady comes into my office" stories abound in veterinary medicine: "Lady comes into my office," says Obenski. "Her dog, wheezing and breathing badly, is dying of congestive heart failure, so we give her these blue pills containing hormones and tell her the dog is not going to live long. So we are surprised when, a month later, she comes back for more blue pills, and we are even more surprised a month after, when she returns for another refill. On her third visit, I said, 'But this dog was at death's door!' And the woman replies: 'The dog actually died a week after you saw it. But during that week he was always trying to make love to the cat. So ever since the dog died, I put one of these pills in my husband's coffee every morning.' "

"Lady comes into my office," Obenski continues, "with a cat with leukemia." The cat is euthanized on the spot, and the lady requests that Obenski store the cat in the freezer for a while. "She telephones the office two weeks later and she says, 'I'm ready to pick up my cat. Let's thaw him out.' The lady had read that freezing kills leukemia virus. So she put two and two together . . . and got five."

D.V.M. put up prizes for the best stories, judged by Obenski: All were published in the magazine. Richard Forrest of Essex Junction, Vermont, was awarded first prize, an airline ticket to the veterinary conference of his choice in the continental United States. Forrest's story concerned an elderly client, Madame X, and her two Chihuahuas, Chico and Maria. Madame X was constantly dressing her dogs in different outfits: Toreador and Spanish dancer, Swiss lederhosen and dirndl dress, ballerina tutu and jacket with tights—the combinations were endless. One morning, a hysterical Madame X burst into Forrest's office, with Chico yelping loudly in her arms. "Chico is in horrible pain!" she yelled. Today, Chico was dressed in a farmer motif: straw hat, gingham shirt and blue coveralls with shoulder straps, decorative rivets, and a zipper down the fly area.

Sobbing, choking, and trying to talk at the same time, Madame X held Chico's head so that he wouldn't bite as Dr. Forrest attempted to conduct an examination. Chico was writhing and crying uncontrollably—until Dr. Forrest unbuttoned the shoulder straps of Chico's coveralls and pulled down the zipper of his fly, which had snagged on the dog's sheath. But this discovery was only the beginning of Dr. Forrest's story. The moment Dr. Forrest released the zipper, Chico gave a loud shriek, urinated on the table and released a load of loose stool. Before Forrest could clean up the mess, Madame X, who had been sobbing throughout the ordeal, began choking, gagging, and coughing.

Then suddenly Dr. Forrest saw the upper plate of Madame X's false teeth shoot from her mouth and land in the midst of the stool-and-urine-laden table. Forrest reached for a towel to clean off the teeth, but Madame X was faster. She dug into the mess of urine and stool, grabbed her teeth and thrust them back into her mouth. Forrest was stunned, but tried his hardest to look away from Madame X's mouth and ignore what had just happened by calming Chico down and explaining to the woman the source of the pain. But Madame X was absolutely ecstatic. "Thank you, thank you, doctor," she said. "You're so wonderful, I could kiss you!" Before he could move—or even think—Madame X's hands were on his cheeks, and she was kissing him full on the lips.

# NEW BOLTON

M ess, dirt, and hard labor are integral parts of the vet-erinary life. At the University of Pennsylvania's New Bolton Center near the Andrew Wyeth Museum in Chester County, veterinarians walk the cutting edge of technology—in a body shop atmosphere. Most of the equipment in the six-hundred-acre complex, which treats twenty-two thousand patients annually, including llamas, goats, pigs, and bongos, the biggest large animal caseload in the country, has been manufactured to industrial specifications.

Here, veterinarian Wendy Vaala is bottle-feeding a hundred-pound, week-old foal that she calls "Tug," its fuzzy, delicate, oblong head tucked tightly under her armpit, a procedure called the "udder bump." Foals eat 20 to 30 percent of their hundred-pound body weight each day. Tug's mom died during childbirth, but Vaala has convinced the owner to lease a $1,900 rent-a-mom to stay with Tug until he's weaned.

Dr. Vaala mops the urine puddled on the rubber pad of Tug's stall. She produces a pile of clean Mickey Mouse sheets from a storage cabinet, changes the sheet on Tug's mattress, and then moves quickly down to the adjacent stall. Even in the neonatal intensive care unit (NICU), a four-million-dollar facility, the work is labor-intensive and often somewhat primitive, with physicians performing basic care tasks a human doctor wouldn't even consider.

The similarities between high-tech human medicine and high-tech veterinary medicine are especially apparent in this unit, with incubator/respiratory hookups, oxygen, suction, and a padded and heated floor. But the traditional doctor/nurse/orderly hierarchy is not as distinct when doctors are mopping urine and shoveling poop. As she mops, she also conducts a nonstop monologue with Tug about her life and his. In fact, as I roam about this veterinary center, I frequently overhear doctors or nurse-technicians discussing medicine, politics, life—whatever—with horses.

Rudy, the copper-colored foal next to Tug, with Elasticron bandages wrapped around its spindly, delicate legs, is a "dummy foal." Burdened with neurological problems, "dummy foals" are often born prematurely; some are blind, can't think clearly or walk. "But that doesn't mean that they can't be saved, that we can't bring them back. One of our favorite dummies we called 'Lurch' because he couldn't stand straight; he was lurching around everywhere. He went on to win a number of races." But in many ways, Rudy, although a "dummy," is similar to a typical human baby. "He's spoiled rotten," Dr. Vaala says. "He won't give up his pillow or his teddy bear."

Rudy's owner wants to offer him for sale, but he has a deformity in his leg that may or may not have been corrected by a recent surgery. Before buying a horse, owners look for "white hairs," because, when horses are cut, the scar has a tendency to grow back white. A resident unwraps Rudy's surgical bandages, a labor-intensive procedure requiring the resident and three colleagues to lower Rudy to the ground and hold him by sitting gingerly on top of him. Meanwhile, Dr. Vaala is restraining Rudy's jealous and concerned mother, who is whinnying and pacing in the adjacent stall.

Everyone gathers around to examine Rudy's legs. At birth, Rudy had been unable to stand. His legs were so bowed, they collapsed inward anytime he tried to get to his feet. Now they look pretty good, but first the staff must wait for the radiologist to take an X-ray so that Vaala can consult with Rudy's surgeons and then advise the owners as to whether additional surgery will be required.

Dr. Vaala is wearing khakis and a flowered shirt. She has reddish brown curly hair guided by combs into a neat cascade down her back. She's wearing battered white leather tennis shoes, and she looks kind of pale and tired, as if she doesn't get enough sun. As she talks, she has a habit of rubbing her hands together and resting her fingertips on her lips like she's praying, which is when you see how battered her hands are. The hands of most of these women and men—students, technicians, and veterinarians alike—are red, chapped, and ugly. These are people who use mops. They don't glove for most procedures and the horses are kicking, pushing, fighting constantly. Long fingernails would be a burdensome disaster.

As they wait for the radiologist, the staff continues to push themselves on Rudy, who periodically kicks in frustration. Every time they relax and begin to feel relatively certain that Rudy is going to sit still and not move, he suddenly rears up and kicks. While we are waiting, Maryse, a veterinarian from Montreal on a fellowship at New Bolton, is kicked in the back of the head or shoulder three different times. Maryse winces each time, but even when a resident offers help, she refuses to relinquish her position. The radiologist arrives some fifteen minutes later and takes pictures, but Rudy must be held down until the film is developed and reviewed for clarity, just in case more pictures are required. The surgeons will then be summoned for evaluation. From beginning to end, the NICU staff will struggle with (and also caress) Rudy for at least an hour.

This is difficult work, and both emotionally and physically intensive, but the task yields its subtle rewards for people who seek a special satisfaction among the offspring of some of the most magnificent thoroughbred horses in the world. Foals are strikingly youthful and innocent. Since the foals are most often placid, and since the stall is padded with straw and sheepskin and bedding, the staff will enjoy this rare opportunity to sit and talk and pass the time of day and lay their hands on their patient.

This contentment that I have both observed and experienced so frequently in the veterinary milieu is representative of the compassion and healing behaviors inherent in the profession. As they sit and talk quietly, caressing and cooing to the frightened little foal, Rudy and his mother gain security and comfort, while the medical staff experience a rare and special intimacy. A long, comfortable silence settles upon the room, periodically interrupted by beeping monitors, rolling medicine carts, grunting ponies.

The NICU is two stories high; a row of windows near the ceiling on all four walls, plus glass-block windows in each stall, allow sunlight to stream in without distracting the animals. Music plays in the background, usually old-fashioned, but befitting the moment. Currently, Johnny Mathis is crooning, "Wonderful, Wonderful."

The walls are newly painted peach with blue trim. The stalls have attractive and functional wooden sliding doors with light blue peek-a-boo bars. The nurses' station in the middle is blue cinder block and glass. A red monorail on the ceiling transports anesthetized horses in a canvas sling from the surgical suite to the ICU and NICU. At New Bolton, 250 feet of monorail connect treatment areas to the operating rooms. The lights that come down from the ceiling have aluminum hoods over the bulbs to mute the heat. They look like the French fry warming lights at McDonald's. There's a rollaway bed in the middle of the NICU, which, for a while, I thought was for the nurses or students to sleep in, but actually doesn't get used, except during the busy season, in February, March, and April, when many baby foals will require special attention. Most racehorses are bred to be born very early in the year; there's an eleven-month period in which a mare is "in foal." The closer to the beginning of the year the better it is for the owner of a foal with a potential to race, for horses born in the same year will compete against one another. In other words, a colt born in January could be racing against a colt who was born in May; though the former will be much stronger, both are considered two-year-olds. Vaala continually reminds me to come back during that period; "you shouldn't miss the craziness of this place." Last winter, the NICU was confronted with thirty-one high-risk pregnancies over a three-month span.

Foals experience many of the same problems as human infants; Vaala is constantly studying and adapting techniques that are practiced in the pediatric NICU. "We find out what works in a baby and then try to extrapolate with foals." Surfactant, for example, that substance normally produced by the lungs to facilitate breathing, has routinely been administered to premature babies. "Recently, we began administering surfactant to premature foals at the time of birth." Vaala and her staff have also worked with a number of human perinatologists (OB-GYNs) studying how they monitor fetal well-being in the uterus. "We have gone to workshops for women with high-risk pregnancy, learning how to detect fetal movement and fetal heart rate through ultrasound." In people, a similar biophysical profile has been developed; they know what the normal and the high-risk fetus should do during any stage of development. Now they have a biophysical profile of high-risk mares, although Vaala acknowledges certain limits. "When you are monitoring a woman with ultrasound, you see the entire two- or three-pound baby. But when we put the probe on a mare, even with our enlarged machine, we only see part of the foal."

There are also potentially vital new medications that have been adapted for foals, but not officially approved for use in a horse. The drugs, used with the owner's permission, frequently produces remarkable success, especially the new antibiotics. The size of the horse often makes such investments prohibitive, however. An antibiotic for a baby that costs $25 a day would cost $250 in a foal. On the other hand, owners are often willing to invest huge amounts, provided a horse will likely come through the experience in an unflawed state. Horses are unique because the babies are so valuable; most small animals have large litters, whereas horses give birth to only one or two foals at a time. An owner might invest $50,000 or more to breed a mare to a stallion—and then wait eleven months before a foal arrives. For horses bred to compete, flaws of any kind are unacceptable, which accentuates the pressure on the veterinarian. In the end it is not a question of life and death as with most babies; in horse racing, survival is not the objective. The objective is perfection—or as close to it as possible.

A technician named Sean walks into the NICU to deliver medications. He begins playing with Tug, who suddenly bursts awkwardly out of his stall in excitement. Sean then decides to mimic Tug, walking like Tug, swinging himself back and forth in an unsteady and comic manner. The nurses who have been caring for foals in adjacent stalls stop, one by one, and begin to watch and laugh as Sean and Tug play.

At first, Dr. Vaala seems unhappy with the commotion Sean and Tug are causing. She is thirty-nine years old and has now worked eight days running, a minimum of fifteen hours each day. She told me that she had once been married and was considering remarriage "if I ever get the time." On an average day, she arrives at the NICU at seven A.M. "and if I'm leaving by nine P.M., that's usually pretty good." She owns two dogs and two cats.

Dr. Vaala always wanted to work exclusively with horses. A mentor advised her to watch as many normal foals as she could. As a student at Penn, she commuted to a farm in Maryland on weekends and hung around the foaling shed. After graduating, she entered into a mixed practice—small and large animals—for a year. She returned to New Bolton to help design the NICU, but the technology often frustrates her, as she is not always permitted to use the tools at her disposal.

"Money is always a problem; there's usually a ceiling, an end point to what clients are willing to pay. The charge for the unit is seventy dollars a day—more when intensive nursing care is required." Most horses are insured for mortality but not for surgery, medication, or sickness. "Human medical doctors never have to deal with what a patient is worth." James Herriot has observed that money has always been a barrier between the farmer and the veterinarian because of a deeply embedded conviction in many farmers' minds that they know more about their animals than outsiders, and it seems like an admission of defeat to pay someone else to fulfill their own responsibilities. About 10 percent of his clients refused to pay.

Dr. Vaala's hard work, long hours, and unblinking dedication are legendary at New Bolton. The joke about Wendy Vaala is that she never gets visitors at the NICU because she will put them to work. After watching Sean and Tug dance around for a few minutes, however, and listening to the NICU staff laugh and cheer, a smile lights up Vaala's face. She momentarily joins Sean and Tug in the middle of the room and jumps around playfully, tossing her head and swinging her arms before guiding Tug firmly back into his stall. Everybody applauds.

# STALLION RING

U nlike Wendy Vaala, whose interest in animals, especially horses, has been a lifetime motivating factor
professionally and personally, Sue McDonnell, an animal behaviorist at New Bolton, began her career in human psychology, but
soon recognized the potential of studying stallions, especially in
the area of sexual dysfunction. The stallion's penis is nearly
identical to the human penis.

This is why the Neuro Science Institute of the National Institutes of Health (NIH), with the National Institute of Diabetic
and Kidney Diseases, funded Dr. McDonnell's investigations:
An increasing number of male diabetics are becoming impotent.
Conceivably, McDonnell's success in regenerating the sexual
lives of thoroughbred stallions might someday impact upon
diabetics.

It seems that stallions are masterful masturbators. A stallion experiences a spontaneous erection and a flexion of the penis—it draws it up against his belly and stimulates itself—about every ninety minutes. Masturbation occurs almost from birth through adulthood, even for castrated stallions, although the interval between masturbation episodes lengthens after castration. "With a video camera, you can get very quantitative about the number of bounces per episode, the duration of the episodes, the intervals between episodes, so it's a nice model for looking at things that might enhance ejaculation," says McDonnell, who has discovered and helped develop medications that will sometimes trigger immediate ejaculation.

A plain-looking woman of forty-three, mother of one child, McDonnell discusses her subject with quiet authority. "I used to talk about my work at cocktail parties, but to the general public, some of the stuff we do seems pretty crude. So I don't say much anymore." She pauses, shrugs, and swivels around in her tiny office, looks me in the eye and asks with enthusiasm, "Do you know how horses breed?" Sensing that she was going to tell me no matter what I said, I did not answer.

"At a certain time of year, males of most animals in the wild, such as deer and antelope, come together and fight it out. The winners get the females. The male horse, in contrast, has a harem, a group of mares, five to ten in number, whom he guards and serves, year-round. The leftover males in the herd travel together in 'bachelor bands,' in which members look after one another.

"But what happens when 'harem stallions' become old and debilitated and lose the ability to keep the harem together—or simply, suddenly, fall off a cliff?" McDonnell asks, pausing briefly. "Within minutes, a bachelor will rise up from the band to become the new harem stallion. You would think all hell would break loose, that these guys would fight to the death to get to the mares, but not usually. Mostly it's like 'Hey, poor old Joe just fell off the cliff. So Frank, it's your turn. Good-bye.' "

To understand this behavior, McDonnell and her colleagues have established a model horse community with Shetland pony stallions. In this controlled atmosphere, researchers can remove the harem stallions one after another, in order to analyze how those chosen differ from other bachelor band members. In the process, they have uncovered one fascinating mystery. As soon as the lowly bachelor band horse becomes the esteemed harem stallion, he experiences tremendous endocrine changes. "His testosterone levels go through the ceiling. But then, guess what happens when the reigning harem stallion is replaced by his predecessor." McDonnell raises and wags a finger. "The harem stallion who has been abruptly relieved of command accepts his demotion without question, trots across the pasture with his tail between his legs, and rejoins the bachelor band."

"And what about his testosterone levels?" I ask.

"Rock bottom almost as soon as he loses his job as harem stallion," McDonnell says.

Later, as we stroll through the pasture assigned to her group on the New Bolton campus a mile from her laboratory, three or four of the Shetlands approach us, swelling their chests and nudging us with their noses. These are the harem stallions. We can literally manipulate their actions. As we move toward the group of mares for which they are responsible, the harem stallions will noisily puff their chests and position themselves in between us and their mares. As we move away from the group, they will abandon us and slowly work their way back to a pivotal position of watchful authority over their herd.

Learning enough about harem stallions and bachelor bands so that behavior might actually be manipulated is McDonnell's primary objective, especially when such knowledge might someday be applied to human problems and concerns. For example, in some of her newest research, McDonnell has discovered that the elevated testosterone levels in harem stallions increases the size of the accessory glands (the prostate, etc.), all of which affects the production of semen and makes the stallions more functional—an unbelievable concept to some people, especially men." In the ultraconservative equine community, the notion that the social environment could alter anatomy has been shocking to those with whom she has shared her preliminary results. "These people [owners and trainers] think 'a horse is a horse is a horse'; you put them on a track, they race; in the barn, they reproduce."

When university president Judith Rodin recently visited New Bolton Center, she ended up in McDonnell's laboratory watching as McDonnell measured the accessory glands of a harem stallion using ultrasound; the stallion's prostrate was filling the screen. Rodin, a behavioral scientist, was fascinated, while the male entourage conducting the tour seemed uncomfortable and perplexed. "They were all standing there amazed that she wanted to keep on looking, and I made a bad joke by remarking, 'I suppose there's a lesson in this for you.'"

The chairman of her department insisted that she elaborate. "Well, if you want to have a smaller prostate, you need to limit your exposure to women and your dominance over other men."

Neither the dean nor the chairman considered her observation particularly funny, but McDonnell was serious. "If low libido, low sperm count, low testosterone were a problem in a man, and with no other sign of any other physical difficulty, I would suggest that he get as much exposure to women as possible. I think it probably would perk things up."

All of this information about horses' masturbation and breeding habits is relatively new and not completely accepted in the veterinary community. Even today, some trainers and veterinarians routinely punish stallions for masturbating, almost as if the stallion were wasting sperm that might otherwise be utilized in the money-making procedure of breeding. There are more than forty U.S. patents for devices specifically designed to inhibit masturbation in horses.

This is what had happened to a prize stallion that had been referred to McDonnell from Cornell School of Veterinary Medicine in Ithaca, New York. Sue McDonnell first saw the horse we'll call "Sunday" on a videotape sent to the University of Pennsylvania's Stallion Reproduction Laboratory, a referral from an animal behaviorist at Cornell. She watched with interest as Sunday mounted, inserted, and thrusted with any mare and with great enthusiasm, but failed to ejaculate. An entire year went by until McDonnell was officially called in on the case.

Someone had decided that the reason the horse was not ejaculating was because he was wasting his virility in the act of masturbation. Thus, a stallion ring, a restricting band constructed of plastic or stainless steel that pinches when the penis becomes rigid, was installed on the horse's penis. In Brazil and Argentina, a second device is sometimes also installed around the horse's belly made of thick brush bristles or jagged nails to inhibit masturbation.

Obviously, injuries are caused by stallion rings and other behavior-restricting devices. Even when the majority of veterinarians considered stallion rings acceptable, which was not too many years ago, the recommendation was always to remove the ring and wash and examine the penis regularly. On this horse, Sunday, the fact that a stallion ring was installed was never reported. The ring became ingrown and invisible. When McDonnell examined the horse, she noticed a ring of scar tissue on the penis and immediately suspected that a ring had been implanted. This was confirmed later by the owners and trainers who, oddly enough, had never made the connection between the stallion ring and impotency. The ring was so deeply embedded that it had to be surgically removed.

A veterinary cardiologist subsequently discovered a thrombosis in the aorta that inhibited 75 percent of the circulation to the genital tissues, which was probably why Sunday initially wasn't ejaculating. But then, psychological trauma set in; McDonnell prescribed pharmacologic agents she had developed. Now the horse is breeding successfully in his own harem without help.

Artificial insemination is prohibited in thoroughbred horses; the horse must mount, insert, thrust, and ejaculate. But even though standardbred horses can be artificially bred in modified situations, sexual dysfunction frequently occurs, often triggered by human error. McDonnell remembers a very high-strung standardbred stallion, previously a good breeder, whose unpredictable, temperamental nature forced owners to tranquilize him frequently, especially while in transport. Horses drop their penises when tranquilized. In this case, the horse was not carefully observed. "The horse got a 'paraphimosis,' which means that from dropping down, his penis became swollen, filled with blood, and lost most of the function. So we have a stallion, a retired champion racehorse, who can't get an erection and has a penis that's kind of puffed up and dangling in outer space all of the time. But, he's got two testicles, and he's probably got great sperm, so now what?"

Upon examination, McDonnell discovered that some good healthy tissue remained high up at the base of the penis. "If you touched this tissue, the horse was willing to thrust. We worked with this horse, and we were able to get him to ejaculate by stimulation of his healthy tissue. We then trained the horse to mount and to thrust, at which point we manually inserted the penis into the vagina and held it in position for ejaculation."

This was a difficult and dangerous task, considering the spirited nature of the horse, which had necessitated the tranquilizer in the first place. "We don't lift horses who cannot mount—they are far too heavy—but we have had horses supported through a sling and then stimulated while they stand on the ground. We might also have people support the horse by standing on both sides to stabilize it." As the horse is having an erection, clinicians manually stimulate the penis. "We rig up a collection device, a plastic bag with a makeshift Velcro seal, like a condom over the penis. You can imagine the sight when they thrust into your hand."

I asked McDonnell the reasons for her choice of scientific specialization; there aren't many people in medicine who dedicate their lives to a stallion's penis. "That's an interesting question; I wonder about it myself," she said. "Next week we are hosting a meeting for people throughout the world interested in erection and ejaculation, and it takes large groups like that to help me realize there's not something inherently wrong with me—unless there's something wrong with all those other people who will be at the meeting with me.

"But I get a kick out of how many people are generally interested in this topic because they have their own problems—secretly. Every time I give a speech at a veterinary school, veterinarians will invariably ask what the human doses might be for the drugs I use for horses." On the surface it may sound eccentric and bizarre, but it is incredible how many people—from all walks of life—are hungry for details and descriptions. Even the most confident and seemingly virile veterinarians will often take a sudden interest in her work, McDonnell has observed.

# INVASIVE PROCEDURES

O rthopedic surgeons in human medicine and equine surgeons in veterinary medicine seem to occupy a similarly elite position in their fields. Mostly men, they are usually athletic in appearance and well-compensated for their work. On a personal level, they are often aloof, seemingly unaffected by the normal drama of life and death in a hospital environment. That's not to say that orthopedic surgeons either in equine or human medicine are not sensitive and caring people, but they will often mask concern and emotion with a forced and arrogant bravado, a behavior I frequently witnessed observing Dr. Dean Richardson.

"Did you kill that foal?" Richardson asks Lance Bassage as we enter the newly constructed postmortem (morgue) facility at New Bolton Center.

Dr. Richardson actually means, "Did you put it to sleep—did

you euthanize it?" But surgeons seem to find a certain comfort in machismo—exaggerating failure or disappointment in themselves or others, ostensibly to lighten the burden of it. Machismo is especially prevalent in relations between senior surgeons like Richardson, a forty-year-old associate professor, and Bassage, a surgical resident.

Enduring callousness is a test of a young surgeon and a rite of passage. One of the most distressing incidents I observed during research for my book about organ transplantation is when an internationally prestigious liver transplant surgeon asked a young surgeon from Australia whose pediatric patient had bled to death on the operating table, "Why did you murder that kid?"

But Richardson might not have understood the special interest that Bassage had taken in the foal. Bassage had persuaded the owner to invest in umbilical surgery, which was successful, but unfortunately, the foal traumatized his leg while fighting off the effects of anesthesia. It was an unavoidable and not uncommon occurrence. I had talked with Bassage about the tragedy of the foal. Bassage is a tall, slender young man with a smooth and wrinkle-free face. "This is a real bugger," Bassage had said, near tears. "Who was to know that the horse would end up hurting himself?" Now, facing Dr. Richardson, he smiled and nodded, masking any of the emotion he had revealed the previous day. "It's been in the cooler all night."

Richardson says he wants a piece of cartilage from the foal's knee to use for research. Bassage presses some buttons on the wall that activate the motor of the monorail that circles the morgue. The chrome doors of the cooler open automatically, and the horse is conveyed to the middle of the room and then lowered to the newly painted blue floor, at Richardson's feet. All around, there are pieces of horse body parts scattered about, on hooks, on tables, and on the floor.

A handsome muscular man, flippant and high-strung like the

thoroughbreds on whom he operates, Dean Richardson stoops down, lifts the foal's injured leg and begins to manipulate it. "The kneecap is broken off, held on by a piece of cartilage. You can flap it like a lid of a plastic container." He looks up. "This is a good example of something you can fix in a human, but the problem is, as this foal has demonstrated, a horse won't sit still long enough to allow itself to heal."

Postmortem is the end of the line for the animals at New Bolton—the last stop on the high-tech monorail of recovery or death. Many horses are actually euthanized on the grass behind this building and then transported unceremoniously with a fork-lift through the two-story-high doors for autopsy. About half of the animals who die at New Bolton are autopsied, a gory prospect for those who are squeamish. But veterinarians and MDs, scientists to the core, are usually energized by the prospect of learning why a patient died and the route a disease traveled. Information gleaned during a postmortem may shed enough light on the mysteries of surgery, biology, and bacteria to make a difference for another patient in the future.

I've always understood the importance of the autopsy, but the day I observed in the temporary postmortem facility in an old garage-barn some weeks before the new facility was completed was quite horrifying. Medical students were deeply involved in an anatomical quest of search and discovery with a half-dozen dead horses in different stages of dismemberment. The sticky incense of burning bone permeated the room. Bone dust created by the power tools used to separate the larger parts of the horse from the carcass wafted up, mixing with splattered blood and congealing into a red paste that seemed to cling to everyone, everywhere. We pulled plastic covers up over our boots and coveralls and slogged around in the paste for the afternoon.

I've witnessed the goriest of surgeries, including heart and lung transplantation, in which the heart and both lungs are lifted, en bloc, from a human chest, revealing a deep crater of bloody nothingness. But there seemed to be purpose in this devastation—an extension of life, combined with a scientific mission. Here, I found the sight of blood and bone, horse heads and assorted body parts scattered about, disgusting; I felt compassion for the students, whose dreamy and idealistic visions of the veterinary lifestyle were undoubtedly violated by this postmortem rotation in a Chicago stockyardlike setting. I muttered excuses about a need to make some telephone calls and exited. One of the benefits of being a writer and not a physician is that I can understand and appreciate my subjects without having to cut them up in little pieces to see inside their bodies or their psyches—at least not literally.

Meanwhile, Dr. Richardson is now attempting to persuade a student to return to New Bolton for an internship, but she declines. "I thought you were interested in horses?" he said.

"That was then," the student answered. "This is now."

"Don't tell me you want to become a dog plumber," said Richardson, sneering.

Richardson glances at his watch, suddenly remembering he is pressed for time. He's got to go to radiology to view X rays of his next case. "So, Dean, you want me to whack off a leg," Lance Bassage calls after him, "or what?"

Initially, Richardson had intended to insert a screw in the knee of his next case, a standardbred three-year-old, but an examination of the most recent X rays reveals that the horse is more damaged than he had originally perceived. He phones the person listed on the chart as owner. Under the circumstances, Richardson suggests to the man on the other end of the line that an entire slab of bone in the left knee must be removed.

"He's seriously damaged goods," Richardson says calmly but crisply into the telephone, squinting down at the film. "And even if you do the surgery, the other knee has to be 'scoped' [arthroscopic surgery] as well. Under the best of circumstances, this horse is going to be out of action a minimum of six months, with only a fifty-fifty chance of ever running again."

Now there is silence. Richardson stares at the horse's chart, flipping pages noisily, nodding and listening. He may be flippant and cynical, but Richardson is well-respected not only for his skill as a surgeon, but his straightforward no-nonsense, honest approach. You may not like what Dr. Dean Richardson tells you, but you can be certain that it will be accurate to the best of his considerable abilities.

After answering a few more questions, Richardson hangs up the phone. The owner can't make a decision because he has to contact his partner. Most horses Richardson works on are business investments, sometimes worth one million dollars or more. Some owners are more caring and compassionate than others, but the bottom line in a decision of this nature, which requires the influx of funds, is whether money will be made—or lost—as a result of the investment. "The objective is to make a profit with the horse—not a friend," Richardson said.

In many cases, surgeons and other VMDs at New Bolton never meet or even converse with the owners; trainers, other veterinarians, or business managers are just as likely to be the contact and decision-making personnel. If hobnobbing with the blue bloods of the horse world is something to which a veterinarian aspires, then they will probably have to buy their own horses to race after all because that is the only way they will truly become an integral part of the "horsy" set.

While waiting for the owner to make a decision, Richardson contacts the referring veterinarian, who reveals his suspicions that the trainer, in charge of the horse on a daily basis, has long been injecting cortisone into the damaged leg to keep the horse running. From the standpoint of both employment (keeping his job) and reputation, the trainer has as much to lose in the racing profession as the owner. Very often, as an inducement, the trainer will retain a financial interest in the horse. Also, as a matter of course these days, trainers and/or owners frequently doctor their own animals. Many medicines used for animals are available to the general public. In horse circles, black market activity in drugs like anabolic steroids has led to many jail sentences through investigation by the Drug Enforcement Agency (DEA) or the USDA.

Not unexpectedly, the conversation with the referring veterinarian makes Richardson angry. He slams the phone down. "This is hideous," he announces. He repeats the word "hideous" to anyone in listening distance in radiology, mostly colleagues, who nod their heads in agreement.

"Some owners . . . ," he tells me, hesitating. Pausing and rephrasing his words, he continues: "Standardbreds will usually make most of their money the first three years in racing. This horse is already three, and he will be out of action for six months after the surgery—dead minimum." In a recent study of 150 horses in which a similar procedure was attempted only 50 percent returned to racing.

In a few minutes, the owner is back on the telephone, having conferred with his partner. "How much will the surgery cost?" he wants to know.

Richardson consults a chart. "A little under two grand."

He pauses and listens as the owner asks additional questions. "Doing nothing is hopeless, as far as racing is concerned," Richardson replies. "Doing surgery is a long shot." He listens again, this time for a longer period. "Look," he says, "that's not my decision, but those are the numbers. I told you before, it's a long shot."

Once again, the owner has something to say; Richardson is silent. Then he shakes his head. "You are not going to collect mortality insurance for euthanasia; you are not paying insurance premiums that the horse will race. You are going to collect only if it is killed. Euthanasia on a racehorse because it is not going to race again is not a collectible diagnosis," he repeats. "If the horse dies of colic or something like that, well then it is different." Another pause. "What can I say? The chances are good that you will invest two thousand dollars and the horse will live out the rest of his life eating grass in the field and never compete again."

Richardson slams the receiver down. He has been polite and restrained on the telephone, but his anger explodes in this room. "This is hideous," he repeats. He is about to continue ranting, when he receives another phone call from the owner. "Okay," he says, hanging up the phone.

"So what's up?" a nurse asks.

"Let's do this surgery," he replies.

The horse is given preoperative sedation, and then led into an induction stall, which is also used as the recovery stall after anesthesia. His legs are shaved, and then scrubbed free of straw, dirt, and hair with yellow soap, revealing a plump pink layer of flesh. Specially designed canvas harnesses are slipped over his head and tail and lashed to thick, heavy hemp ropes on six sides. Then the ropes are passed through portholes in the walls and doors of the stall. Each rope will be manned by a member of the surgical or recovery team. Both the walls and the floor of the stall are padded. Horses tend to want to stand up too early after anesthesia, but then frequently bounce off walls and crash to the ground and injure themselves. This is how Lance Bassage's foal was traumatized.

As part of the newest surgical suite, a recovery pool has been installed at New Bolton to minimize this danger. Horses are transported directly from surgery via monorail into a fifteen-thousand-dollar rubber raft, which is then lowered into a deep pool of warm water. When they awake, they can thrash around without hurting themselves or anyone else. When fully alert and in control, the horse is lifted out of the water. The canvas harnesses are untied. Recovery pools are very new, however, and most horse inductions and recoveries still take place in an induction/recovery stall.

Now a "code four" is announced over the intercom, which will summon enough manpower to protect the horse during induction. Three veterinary students soon arrive; one man and two women to help with the ropes. The remaining ropes are manned by the anesthesiologist and veterinary technicians.

A muscle relaxant is injected into the horse by anesthesiologist Kim Olsen. Soon the horse begins to sway back and forth, and then sinks to the ground. Just at that point—a bare second in limbo prior to a free-fall collapse—the ropes are crisply drawn inward, catching and holding him in midair. A motor kicks in. Heavy chains are lowered from an electric hoist on the monorail and attached to the canvas harness. The motor kicks in a second time, and the horse is lifted high off the ground and carried swiftly into the operating suite, where it is lowered onto a specially designed operating table with removable pieces to accommodate different-sized animals, including cows and llamas. Breathing devices for horses and humans are basically the same—except for size, perhaps a ten to one ratio. The ventilator tubing is identical to that of a large Shop Vac. The staff has fifteen to twenty minutes for intubation, meaning connection to anesthesia. Through the entire procedure, Olsen, a DVM from the University of Minnesota who has been at New Bolton for the past seven years, keeps up a constant banter with her patients.

"I have worked at human hospitals, and I don't like to be around sick people. And fortunately here a lot of our patients are not sick. They are healthy athletes with fixable problems. To me, it's much easier to like a horse patient than a human patient. I find all animals easy to like. Cows, sheep, horses are so magnificent and wonderful. It always surprises me how easy they are to work with and how cooperative, especially considering the fact that they really don't know what it is you are doing to them and why you are hurting them so badly." As to why she chose such a behind-the-scenes job as anesthesiology: "Lots of people want to be surgeons. But not a lot of people want to be anesthesiologists. The gratification is more a mental thing, much more of an intellectual, problem-solving endeavor."

A gigantic caulking gun is utilized to cleanse the horse's mouth of hay and other debris. "Horses are easy to intubate," a technician tells me. The horse's tongue is pressed flat against a mouthpiece that has been slipped down into his throat. Tubes twice the width of a garden hose extend from the ventilator to the mouthpiece. The ventilator sounds like an air pump in a gasoline station. It provides the horse with six to seven breaths a minute. Meanwhile, an EKG is taken, and the horse's blood will be monitored through a catheter sunk in an artery. The horse's rear legs are lashed down to the surgery table with heavy leather straps. The front legs—the surgical fields—are belted down at the front of the table on pegs with pads called "erector sets" because of the easily adjustable way in which they fit together. Next comes an alcohol, or "white glove," prep to make certain the surgical field is sterile.

Everyone in this room is female, except for me and Richardson, a revealing mirror of the future of the profession. "At night, when we do surgical emergencies we're sometimes staffed completely by women," a resident says. "No men on campus, except for security. It is getting to the point that there are so many women coming into the profession that men are starting to get special preference for certain positions."

During surgery, Dean Richardson is ever more hyper and impatient. He works fast and has a great facility for concentration. After scrubbing, gowning, and gloving, he feels around the surgical field with his thumb, and then grabs a scalpel, while directing a nurse to beam the spotlight on the point of incision. He cuts quickly, no ceremony or hesitation. Blood spurts out, dripping on the drape and onto the floor. He digs into the flesh and muscle with an instrument resembling a screwdriver. Soon comes the sound of metal scraping against bone and cartilage.

What always surprises me about surgery is how jerky and ungraceful it is—and simultaneously how automatic; there are frequent opportunities for creativity in surgery, but mostly it is done by rote. A good surgeon must have good hands and a strong constitution to prepare for the intense pressure of long and focused procedures. But more than anything else, a surgeon must possess the facility of perfect imitation—duplicating a procedure he or she might have witnessed dozens or even hundreds of times—while being ready to respond with instinctive, intelligent abandon in unexpected emergency situations. Meanwhile, the patient, in this case a horse, lies on the erector-set table, eyes open, tongue wrapped around mouthpiece, asleep and oblivious.

Richardson digs and fights and twists for a long time. Once in a while he grunts or groans, until finally unearthing his prey—a chunk of bone the size of a quarter, about a quarter-inch thick. Soon he discovers another piece of bone, smaller. "It's hard to believe that this horse could walk at all with those chunks of bone floating around inside of him—let alone race!" Richardson comments. "The owner is doing this surgery because he paid a lot of money for this horse and so far hasn't gotten much in return." He pauses. "That's his business . . . I guess."

"What do you think?" a resident asks as Richardson examines the slab of bone that he has removed.

"The knee will never be the way God made it," Richardson replies. "But it will hold up if the horse has guts." He pauses to study the bone, held tightly in a clamp, then adds: "Although the trainer says that the horse has no guts whatsoever."

"He's a very sweet horse," the anesthesiologist says.

"Which means that the trainer is probably right, and he has no guts whatsoever," Richardson replies. "Last thing the owner wants is a very sweet horse. You want your racehorse to be aggressive."

Orthopedic surgery is not always the answer when a horse loses its ability to race at full speed or its will to gallop aggressively and win, Richardson admits; in fact, surgeons at New Bolton have developed a number of highly sophisticated diagnostic tools in order to understand the often subtle and complicated reasons why horses experience difficulty on the racetrack.

# THE QUITTER

The horse Eric Parente has been asked to evaluate is a quitter. This horse goes like hell for five-sixths of the race and then, just about the time the owners are counting their money and computing their profits, he slows down. Parente, a thirty-three-year-old veterinarian, a graduate of Cornell School of Veterinary Medicine, whose specialty is sports medicine, is muscular and well-built, with thick brown hair lightly speckled with gray, a square jaw, and a row of perfect teeth. His office is a mess. There are sweat clothes and running shoes stashed under his desk. He's wearing basketball shoes, white socks, khakis, a light-blue shirt with a New Bolton emblem on it, significantly wrinkled after a long semisleepless night.

Among other interests, Parente has been focusing his attention upon the many problems having to do with lameness in the hock, which is a common ailment for horses. Hocks are like human ankles. Steroids are usually used to treat these problems, Parente says. "The cheaper horses get more steroids because they're not going to win many races, so the owners race them and forget them, whereas for a more expensive horse an owner will invest the money to permanently heal the lameness and eradicate the pain."

As we walk from his office to the Jeffords Treadmill Facility, Parente points out that 50 percent of the horses that are bred for racing never get to the track. But in this case, the chocolate brown three-year-old with a brown mane and one white foot races well until he slows at the home stretch, the point at which he should be barreling at top speed. Preliminary examination has ruled out obvious problems, such as lameness.

First, Parente must grind off the traction-inducing toe grabs on the horse's shoes, which would tear into the rubber of the treadmill. For this he utilizes a large carpenter's sander with extra-coarse sandpaper. He shows the grinder to the horse and triggers it so that the horse can become familiar with its sound—and also learn to trust him. He also places his hand on the horse. He holds on when the horse tries to jerk away. In a persistently gentle manner, Parente holds on tightly until the horse is comfortable with his touch.

I've observed him practice a similar philosophy with the horse's mouth during a dental examination. "Hold on, allow them to make their objections. But be relaxed and firm at the same time," he says. Horses, Parente explained, have incisors in front and molars in the back of the mouth, and an interdental space in the middle. "So if your psychology fails, and they decide to bite down with your hands in their mouth, your fingers will be safe if you keep them in the interdental space." As an added safeguard, a veterinarian can reposition a horse's tongue to the side so that it lies between molars. "Then, if they do get testy and chomp down, it will be on their own tongue, and they will be in much more pain than you. In that way, you can examine one side of the mouth in relative safety. Then flip the tongue back to the other side of the mouth and complete your examination."

Now Parente slowly creeps under the horse, lifts its front leg at the hock, and begins to grind. The noise is disturbing to the horse, as are the fiery metal sparks, which he carefully directs away from any contact with the horse. Leg coverings have been wrapped around the horse below the knee, but despite the three students holding and attempting to keep the horse relatively still, it rears up and kicks, a hoof whizzing past Parente's shoulder as he jumps away.

They try again. This time they employ a tool made of an ax handle with a loop of clothesline at the end. The loop is fitted around the horses's nose, and the ax handle is twisted until the horse is rendered under control. It's called a twitch, as in, "Do you want me to 'twitch' him, Dr. Parente?"

After the grinding, the horse is allowed to become accustomed to the treadmill by walking around it, sniffing and nudging it with his nose. Then he is led up the ramp and onto the matted rubber floor; eventually he is tethered up against a breastplate. The speed of the running surface is controlled from a console.

The treadmill simulates racing conditions. At a top speed of thirty-seven miles per hour, its running surface is elevated to an uphill slope of six degrees, which forces animals to work harder. For diagnostic procedures, the animal is worked up to 200 to 240 heartbeats per minute, the heart rate at racing speed. In the process, sports medicine clinicians compile an impressive broadside of tests, including cardiovascular evaluation utilizing a radio telemetric heart monitor. An endoscope, inserted into the horse's throat through a nostril, reveals the larynx, viewed on a large TV screen to detect irregularities that may shed light on the "noisy breathing" of a racer, a sign that a horse's airway is somehow being restricted.

Other crucial measurements compiled while the horse is running include oxygen consumption, $CO_2$ and lactic acid production, respiratory and upper airway flow, blood and venous pressures, blood gases, glucose metabolism, and oxygenation. These measurements are fed into three computers, located in the diagnostic laboratory adjacent to the treadmill. In addition to two stalls, the centerpiece of the building is a twelve-windowed steeple braced by two magnificent arches that rise dramatically to the ceiling. "It's kind of like the Sistine Chapel," Parente says.

The treadmill, made by Walmanik International Corporation in Freedom, Pennsylvania, is fully enclosed by bullet-proof polycarbonate in case a horse loses a shoe while galloping. Perhaps a thousand standardbred and thoroughbred horses have been evaluated on this treadmill since the diagnostic center opened in 1992. "I guess you could find out what's wrong with this horse, sooner or later, by trial and error, but the investment in time and energy might be prohibitive," Parente says.

Now the treadmill is activated, allowing the horse to walk, at first slowly and then more briskly. Gradually, the horse is led into a slow and steady trot, lasting just a few minutes. The pace is reduced, then once again increased. This time the horse is worked from a walk to a trot to a canter. It is amusing to observe the horse orient himself to the treadmill. The floor suddenly starts to move beneath him, but he is amazed to discover that the walls are staying right where they are.

The horse steps gingerly on the moving tread, as if attempting to clutch the ground with nonexistent toes. Attendants have been stationed on both sides of the horse to steady and control him with guide ropes. Once in a while, the horse bristles. His pace breaks. A couple of taps on the rear with a crop by one of the attendants reminds him to resume his unhurried canter.

The space beneath the treadmill is hollow, and the hooves striking the tread make deep, full-timbered drumbeats. As the horse's speed increases, hooves pounding, the intensity infects everybody gathered in the complex, students, observers, and clinicians alike. But before the horse reaches his galloping peak of power, the pace is eased again. The horse is bathed and rested. An hour later, the official test begins.

The horse ran two miles in the warm-up phase, but the test will be about two and a half miles long—and much more intense. While waiting, Parente shows me videotapes of a racing horse's normal breathing rhythm recorded by the endoscope. "Before having the capacity to videotape the epiglottis, veterinarians would interview jockeys about the 'noisy breathing' a horse was making. Or the vet had to sit on a rail and listen as the horse galloped by."

Since joining the treadmill diagnostic team and identifying and repairing breathing problems, which has become a special interest, Parente has had one horse achieve a lifetime speed mark. "I look at the newspaper from time to time to see who's racing, and I often recognize the names of the winners as a horse I worked on. That's a great payback."

Another payback is closer to his heart: As a young boy, Parente's father spent a great deal of time at the racetrack with a favorite great-aunt. Inspired by his father's stories, Parente chose veterinary medicine as a career and equine surgery as a specialty, even though he seldom rides. Even now, six years out of veterinary school, he suspects he hasn't been in the saddle ten times in his entire life. His father is uncomfortable leading a horse on a leash. But Parente, his father, brother, and mother are not the least bit uncomfortable buying and racing thoroughbred horses.

The family started with a five-thousand-dollar cheap claimer and is now involved in the upper echelon of horse racing known as "stakes racing" as owners of a two-year-old thoroughbred whose grandfather is the famed triple-crown winner Seattle Slew. Their thoroughbred's father is named "Houston." The Italian word for aunt is "Zia," and Parente's father's nickname for his favorite great-aunt was Ziz. Thus the name, "Tex Ziz Slew." Parente, who is engaged to an equine veterinarian he met at Cornell, is happy with his work and life. "The horses are athletes, and the challenge physical and intellectual. You try to finesse rather than overpower the animal. To me, that's what racing and training is all about."

Soon "the quitter" is brought back onto the treadmill. The breastplate at the front of the horse is removed. When horses reach a full gallop, they sometimes get so carried away that they want to try to jump over the breastplate. Now everyone gathers around, positioning themselves in front of a monitor. Then an attendant steps forward, placing the twitch on the horse as Parente inserts the endoscope tube into the nostril for the video-tape of the throat. Now the twitch is removed. The treadmill elevation is increased three degrees. The horse walks, trots, canters—and then explodes into a sustained gallop.

Against the black tread of the floor, the brown hooves are lost in the blur of the horse's gallop; all we can see after a while is the flash of a single white hoof. His mane is bouncing against his neck. The thundering sound is deafening. The horse begins to snort. He is being slapped on the butt with a crop from both sides now. His body is strained. His muscles are flexing. His eyes are glazed over with excitement. A technician is yelling out numbers as she glances back and forth at the heart monitor. A veterinarian visiting from Ohio State University is bellowing, "Hup! Hup!" Someone else begins to yell, "Yahoo!" The scene is hypnotic. Everyone is either screaming or stomping their feet.

Suddenly, at the two-mile mark, something happens. A subtle measure of intensity in the horse seems to dissipate. Did he lose momentum? Did that stallion, that gallant racer, in fact, quit? He is slapped several more times with crops, but clearly something significant has occurred. The treadmill slows down, gradually. The test is over. The veterinarian from Ohio State applauds.

Immediately, Eric Parente goes to the videotape, rewinds and plays it back. "Here's the problem." The horse is displacing his palate, which folds up over the epiglottis and partially restricts breathing. "Listen to the sound," Parente says, turning up the volume. "Hear it? *Huh, huh, huh.* His airway closes down on him from time to time, and he's struggling, can't expire fully, and since he can't expire fully, he also can't get a fresh full swallow of air. So when he breathes in, half of the air he's trying to breathe has already been used. It's all here on the tape," Parente concludes.

I ask if "noisy breathing" is the same as "roaring."

A roarer, he explains, can't open his arytenoid all the way because of fatigue. "When a horse is going full tilt both arytenoids should remain completely open. A horse will 'roar' when one collapses and shuts down." The arytenoid flaps every time the horse breathes in, like the swinging door on a cowboy saloon, which is how the roar is generated. A couple of different surgical procedures are used to help silence the roaring horse, one called a laryngoplasty, which is tying back the arytenoid so that the paralyzed vocal cord is removed from the airway. Sports medicine surgeons at New Bolton will perform about a hundred of these procedures a year.

Officially, the quitter's diagnosis is dorsal displacement of the soft palate. It's a functional problem in the throat, as compared to a structural problem, which means it may be more difficult to repair. Parente will suggest a minor procedure that has been borrowed by veterinarians from pediatric surgeons. For children with aphonia, who cannot trigger enough vibration in their vocal cords to make a noise, a liquid Teflon-like material is injected under the epiglottis. Scar tissue is formed, stiffening the bottom of the epiglottis.

The tool utilized for the procedure resembles a caulking gun with a long needle. Pediatric surgeons inject the Teflon in this way through the mouth with children under anesthesia. "We do it with an incision underneath the larynx. You couldn't ever reach the epiglottis through the horse's mouth. We've had relatively good success with this procedure for horses who 'displace,' " Parente concludes. "This may not be the horse's only problem, but it is a partial answer to the owner's nagging question: 'Why does this horse quit?' "

# DIFFICULT DECISIONS

D
r. Wendy Freeman will frequently refer patients to Eric Parente because of his compassion for horses, whether they be racers or beloved companions and pets. As we talk, Freeman, a veterinarian at the New Bolton Center Field Service, guns the accelerator of her mobile clinic—a large pickup truck with a double cab outfitted with a fiberglass shell with drawers and compartments designed specifically for practicing veterinary medicine. She thunders out of the parking lot and down the road, the oversized rear tires spitting gravel. As she drives, she fingers the stethoscope draped haphazardly around her steering wheel and frequently turns to make eye contact. At first, her lack of attention to driving makes me nervous, but I soon note her uncanny ability to sense dips and turns in the road. Luckily, in this backcountry, there are only occasional

oncoming vehicles, controlled primarily by people who regard driving as an afterthought.

Although she will treat a variety of animals on the many farms that dot this fertile valley, her specialty is "ruminants," sheep and goats especially, for which she possesses a special passion. Ruminants are cloven-hoofed animals, with four compartments in their stomachs; they ruminate, meaning they eat food, regurgitate it back up, and eat it again. "Cows chew their 'cuds'; sheep, goats, deer, elk, moose—most 'food' animals—can eat fibrous plants in this manner and get nutrition from it. Mostly, the diseases they get are straightforward and simple to treat. If they end up having a serious enough disease, you euthanize them, because they're not worth a lot of money."

She shrugs and turns toward me, as if she has said something that might offend. Freeman has a well-scrubbed look: tall, slender, plain. Wearing faded, almost-white khakis, she is lean, freckled, and boyish. "When you work with farm animals, it boils down to economics; you know, a farmer looks at a sick animal and says, 'I can replace her for fifty dollars, why spend five hundred dollars trying to make her better?'"

For ruminants, there is a large but growing minority of owners who treat animals like pets, which makes the veterinarian's work more satisfying and less commercial. And these days, pig owners are becoming increasingly sensitive and sentimental. Veterinarians have been eliminated from day-to-day swine work, such as vaccinations and castrations. Except in emergency situations, most of the pigs that veterinarians deal with these days are pets. Vietnamese pot-bellied pigs are the current rage. "People keep them in their houses, let them sleep in their beds, drive them around in their cars. They're intelligent animals, but difficult. Pigs scream as soon as you grab them, and they don't stop screaming until you let go. So your client is hysterical because their beloved pig is screaming, and they're not sure why you're hurting him; they don't understand that it's normal pig behavior."

Horses, such as the one she will be examining on her first stop that day, frequently generate an emotional attachment that makes an owner more sentimental than financially responsible. Ricki, who lives in a rambling brick ranch house on the edge of a lime green field dotted with a rainbow of summer wildflowers, is clearly perplexed over the fate of a thickset, whiskered twenty-eight-year-old mare named Honey, who is slowly and painfully dying from old age and arthritis.

Listening to Ricki talk about her daughter's unwillingness to even so much as enter into a conversation concerning the euthanasia of Honey and nodding frequently, Freeman removes the plastic cap of a needle by yanking it with her teeth and proceeds to vaccinate Honey for botulism and rabies. Because one hand is always holding down or caressing an animal, veterinarians, as a matter of course, employ their teeth as a third hand.

"Sometimes an old or sick horse like Honey will be 'cast,' that is, fall or lie down to sleep and be unable to lift themselves back up," Freeman tells me.

"We sometimes find her wedged under the pasture gates or the stall door," Ricki says. "But my daughter is twenty-five years old and has never known life without Honey."

Freeman continues down the line of Ricki's three other horses, yanking off the caps of needles with her teeth, patting and caressing each animal with gentle assurance before sinking the needle into a fleshy area at the nape of the neck.

"What do you think we should do about Honey?" Ricki asks.

"It's a quality of life issue," Freeman replies. "Is she eating well, maintaining her weight? Ambulatory? I've seen some very lame horses that still had life quality; they're hobbling, but happy. When you get small animals that are so sick they can't make it outside to go to the bathroom so they're urinating in the house, that's a different issue. Dogs that are house-trained don't like to go to the bathroom in the house; they get upset, they have anxiety attacks. It is very painful and embarrassing for them."

"So do you think it is time she be put to sleep?"

"When you think the time has come, I'll support you. I'll do it here in Honey's home where she feels comfortable or I'll take her away and put her to sleep in the hospital, whatever is easier for you."

"I don't want my horse to become a pasture potato," Ricki says. "What should I do?"

Freeman smiles, but shakes her head in sympathy. "I wish I had ten dollars for every person who wants me to make that decision for them."

On the average, Wendy Freeman will see eight cases a day, treating horses, goats, sheep, cows, and an occasional llama. On an emergency basis, she will be summoned by farmers for dystocias, which are difficult births, and pregnancy toxemia, common in ewes close to lambing—and the walking wounded from dog attacks. For horses, lameness and foot abscesses are common, as is colic—stomach pain. Cows get "milk fever," and when they get into the grain they will often overload, like a child with a stomachache after eating a package of cookies. Overeating could kill any farm animal.

Difficult pregnancies and deliveries are routine and troublesome. "I once chased a beef cow with a newborn calf hanging out of her by its feet. She was running wild in a two-acre field. The farmer and I tried to round her up with our trucks and push her into a shed. We gave up that idea when she smashed in the doors of both trucks with head butts. So we decided to rope her; took us an hour before we got the rope around her. We tied her leg to the bumper of my truck, stretched her out, knocked her down, pulled the calf out. It was rough work."

"Rough work" is an understatement in this particular instance and in calving generally, which is one of the most grueling aspects of her job, especially for a spare, slight woman like this veterinarian, who weighs all of 120 pounds. Sometimes even catching a wild and frightened cow in this bizarre drama is only the beginning. Sometimes a cow is so swollen with pregnancy and the calf wedged so deeply inside the womb that the struggling veterinarian, reaching and groping vainly for hours on end, will lose her sense of time and grip on reality, and eventually begin to imagine the nightmarish possibility of literally losing herself inside the mother. Or sometimes the veterinarian, shivering violently in the freezing night air, drained of all energy and spirit, will begin to envision the unmentionable but tempting notion of failure—of giving up—and the alluring rewards such a decision might bring: warmth, food, coffee, sleep.

But even in triumph, when the calf is finally pulled out, she will often experience a momentary and panicky feeling of failure. Calves in difficult births frequently look dead when they are first born. Their eyes are glassy; their tongues are bloated. The veterinarian knows she must encourage and coax life back, clear throats of possible obstructions, initiate artificial respiration—and pray through agonizingly long seconds until the animals can wrench their sticky eyes open and begin their tentative jerky attempts to communicate to instigate control over their bodies. In the end, the veterinarian says, she always experiences simultaneously fear, exhaustion, and frustration, along with an exhilarating feeling of satisfaction, which she carries with her—until the next long night.

Recently, a cow decided to calve in a swamp two miles away

from the nearest barn and in a pouring rain. The farmer, a stubborn and money-minded businessman, waited until 10:30 P.M. to telephone Freeman. She arrived within thirty minutes, helped hitch the cow to a tractor and drag her to solid ground. "I should say *solid mud*. We were covered in guck. Our rain gear was useless." She tried to deliver the calf, but it was breach, necessitating surgery.

The farmer wanted her to perform surgery in the field. It was the most economical approach, but not the safest for either mother or calf. When Freeman pointed out that they were standing in a driving rain, the farmer suggested pitching a tent. But she countered by stressing the need for electricity, so the farmer said he'd make a skid with the tractor—tomorrow—and take the mother down to the barn. She refused to wait a day for the skid and persisted until the farmer agreed to call for the ambulance from a nearby animal clinic so that the delivery could be made under safer conditions. In the end, her client—the farmer—had been cooperative, but some farmers are more difficult to deal with than their animals. Farmers often think that they know more about their animals than veterinarians do.

A farmer telephoned one night and asked her to do a cesarean on a pregnant mare who was toxic and dying, in order to save the foal. This surgery took place in the field, lighted by the headlights from two pickup trucks. They put a catheter in the mare's neck so that the euthanization could come immediately after delivery, blocked out an area on her stomach, and cut her open. The foal came out easily, but the mare was dead.

"It's pouring down rain, lightning and thunder crackling everywhere. The mare's lying right along a major highway, and I said, 'You have to get this horse out of here. Nobody is going to want to see or smell this dead mare with all of her guts out when the sun comes up." Persisting, Freeman asked why the mare had been so sick in the first place. He was not a regular client; she had never met the man. The farmer said that the horse had been sick for three days, walking kind of funny, not eating well, acting strangely. She then asked the million dollar question: "No," the farmer replied, "she's not been vaccinated for rabies."

At this point, she knew that her dealings with this stubborn farmer were going to become considerably more difficult. "We need to take her head off and check for rabies," she said. "We argued for a while, but I insisted." Reluctantly agreeing, the farmer stepped back to watch. "So now I'm sawing her head off out in the middle of the rain. I finish, stick it in a bucket." Freeman's truck was parked on the other side of a fence dividing the field from the highway. Her plan was to hand the bucket over the fence to the farmer to put it on her truck, but now, suddenly, the farmer was nowhere to be found. So she balanced the bucket on top of the fence so that she could climb over and carry it to where her truck was parked. No sooner did she get on the fence, when the bucket fell over, and the horse's head rolled into the middle of the highway. "I ran like hell, scooped the head up, threw it into my truck and jumped in. Whoever drove by during that whole fiasco probably thought *Godfather* was happening all over again." Fortunately, the animal was not rabid.

Freeman works part-time at a small animal clinic in Delaware. "You go into the clinic, and there's all those little animals, and they're all sick, and they're looking at you with big eyes because you're the person that's going to make them better. So here's a little creature who's dependent on you, like an infant, you know? That's when I know why I'm a veterinarian. You get satisfaction from the animals. It's some people—like that farmer—that give you aggravation."

* * *

Freeman locates a spot in the barn directly beside an electric outlet and plugs in the disbudding iron. She walks outside, opens a pen in which two calves are waiting, selects a brown-spotted calf ("the kind that makes chocolate milk," she jokes) and brings it inside. Working quickly, she shaves the hair from around the horns, and then reaches into her bag for lidocaine, a pain blocker, which she has already siphoned into a hypodermic needle. She injects the lidocaine directly around the horn.

Next comes the electric disbudding iron, which resembles a branding iron, round, like a large "O," not unlike a packaged donut. She grabs the calf's ear, wedges its head against her body, places the "O" of the iron around the calf's horn, and then, bringing the iron slowly downward, digs the hot iron into the calf's little head.

First there is a wisp of bluish white smoke, and then the dank, stark stench of burning fur. Then comes the richer more primeval aroma of roasting skin, followed by the sound of searing bone, as she applies increasing pressure. Pressing into the calf's head with the iron, she twists her wrist back and forth repeatedly until smoking copper-colored rings show through above the ears. It looks as if the smoke is emanating from the calf's head, as if the soul of this tiny helpless animal has suddenly been apprehended by the devil. "The horn is growing from cells within and below the hair, and so if you kill the skin around the horn, there will never be another horn returning. Animals sense the heat, but do not feel any pain," she adds.

In the days of the wide-open range, horns were needed by livestock for protection. Now, horns serve no practical purpose and, in fact, may be used aggressively and cause harm to a farmer's valuable herd. Veterinarians are asked to perform a number of such procedures, including the removal of waddles—appendages of skin that hang down from the necks of goats. For this procedure, she will snip off each waddle with a gigantic clipper, as if she were clipping fingernails. The animal may not experience physical pain, "although losing part of your anatomy can't be particularly pleasant." For cosmetic purposes, veterinarians may also remove the third teat on the developing mammary gland of pygmy goats, which are considered a genetic flaw that disqualifies the goat from competition or breeding. Using a local anesthetic to dull the pain and snipping the teat with a clipper resembling an ordinary pliers, the procedure is completed in three minutes flat.

Disbudding the second calf does not go as smoothly as in the first instance, perhaps because the first calf defecated on the floor during the procedure, and so now the second calf, an emaciated pale white baby of about four months, is slipping around in the feces. As the calf struggles, its flying hooves pepper Freeman's khaki pants with feces and track it on her leather tennis shoes. "They love to stand on your feet," she says. Freeman slips and catches herself on a rail. "It's kinda like ice out here."

Some of the most hazardous moments a veterinarian might experience are caused by fecal matter. Zoo veterinarian Don Neiffer has a scar on his leg from a cut he received while restraining an emu, a large African bird. "I slipped and fell on its feces, and he cut me with his claw." There's a male gorilla who constantly bombards him with fecal matter. "He thinks he's a discus thrower. When the feces hits the cage wires, it spreads out like it was shot from a Vegimatic."

Freeman burns in the disbudding horn, twists it round and round, the calf jumping with each grinding twist. She blows the smoke away from her face. "It would be nice to have a little fan on your shoulder," she says. After the disbudding, she rubs the hot circle of the iron on top of the tiny remaining buds, one at a time, to cauterize them. She sprays the burning circles with yellow antibacterial Furox and returns the calves to their pen. The horns will fall off in a couple of weeks.

Back in the truck, her gear stored neatly in the drawers and cabinets of her traveling veterinary station, Dr. Freeman picks up our conversation, as if the disbudding never occurred or was much too common and ordinary to discuss: "There was a woman at a riding stable where I was working, a schoolteacher. Her horse was old and thin, and very lame; she could no longer ride him. But, every day, she went to that barn and took him for a walk and gave him carrots; she'd always be hanging out and letting him graze. And I would go over and pet him and say, 'Oh, Shadow looks good.' I never left the stable without saying hello or good-bye to Shadow.

"That year, I went away for the Christmas holidays, and while I was gone, Shadow had emergency surgery at New Bolton, and it turned out he was dying. But Pat wouldn't let anybody put him to sleep until I came back. She wanted me to drive to Limerick, a pet cemetery, and euthanize Shadow there so that we could bury him, but by the time I got back, it was too late. He needed to be euthanized immediately. I said, 'Pat, you need to say good-bye; he's suffered enough.'" When Pat walked into the stall and whispered his name, Shadow lifted his head, turned to look at her, and started to nicker. "We all started to cry," she said, "even the surgeon, Eric Parente, if I recall. Later, we loaded the horse on the trailer for her so that she could bury him.

"Not long afterward, the woman sent me a letter about how it meant so much to her that I would say hi to Shadow all the time. I remember reading the letter and thinking, 'Isn't that something? Just me stopping and saying hello to her horse made her feel like he was really important.' Those are the kinds of things that some clients want you to do; some clients want to feel that veterinarians really care about their animal.

"Four days before last Christmas, I had to put an old horse down for a girl that had asthma," Freeman tells me as we arrive back at her office at New Bolton, where she is scheduled to meet her final patient of the day, a goat. "This girl would go to the barn with a little mask on her face every day and take care of that horse. He got real sick the weekend before Christmas; I was on duty, and I was up all night with him for two nights, and he wasn't getting better. She had run out of funds, and we had decided to euthanize him. Even now I can picture that little girl's face, as she walked into the barn with the little mask on and . . . I was the one who had to kill her horse. It was the worst Christmas of my life."

In a few minutes, Freeman is stooping on a patch of grass adjacent to the parking lot near her office, examining a brown Nubian goat inflicted with a rare kidney disease far too expensive for its owner to afford to treat. The goat's owner is a woman with whom she has worked for a half-dozen years who is suffering from an increasingly debilitating case of multiple sclerosis. The conversation is short and to the point; the woman's options are significantly limited. "Okay," she says to the veterinarian, holding her hand like a traffic policeman, palm straightforward, signaling STOP. "That's enough talk."

Looking back, I realize that the euthanasia happened quite quickly, but at the time it occurred, the process seemed agonizingly long. I watched it as if it were being played back to me in slow motion.

Wendy Freeman takes out a catheter with a long tube filled

with pink liquid (sodium phenobarbital) and injects it into the goat's neck. First blood spatters onto her hand from the catheter. For an instant, the little goat seems to simultaneously inflate itself—and momentarily freeze—midair. Then, a silent single shudder ripples like quiet thunder through every dip and graceful curve of her dramatic, biblical body. Finally, the goat caves in, and collapses on the grass with a muffled thud.

Now the woman cries. She sits on the ground and pets her goat, stroking the goat's head and laying each ear, one at a time, on top of the forehead, tears streaming down her wrinkled cheeks. Freeman reaches down and attempts to close the goat's eyes with the palms of her hands. But the eyes open back up again, continuing to assert themselves. Those eyes are ice blue. They look like diamonds or stained glass glinting in the sun.

I don't know if anyone realized what happened at that particular moment. Or why Freeman selected such a public place to perform such a private act. Many people seemed to be going about their day as if nothing had changed, as if an animal hadn't lost a life and a woman, who herself is slowly dying, hadn't lost a friend. On the other side of the grass, a stable hand loading a horse on a trailer is talking loudly to a companion. Maintenance workers drive by, smiling and waving. Daphne, a high school student who has been interning with Freeman, has joined us in our tight little circle of mourning. The goat continues to shudder and groan, the woman stroking its ears.

"He's already dead," the woman says aloud. "Even though he's making these noises, I know they're involuntary. He's not coming back."

Soon the woman struggles to her feet, hobbles back to the road and climbs shakily into her pickup truck. She starts the motor and drives away. I can see her watching us in her rearview mirror. Now Daphne, the veterinarian, and I are standing alone on the grass, staring quietly down at the goat. "It was a nice goat," Wendy Freeman says. "I wanted to tell the woman, 'Let's put her in the hospital and I'll pay the charges to fix her up.' It would have cost three hundred dollars. But I do too much of that; I just didn't want to spend my own money this time."

# Not Just an Ordinary
# Veterinary School Vet

•─────────────────────────•

Farm or food animal work, which is a large part of Wendy Freeman's day-to-day responsibilities in the New Bolton field service, is undoubtedly the most difficult, physically exhausting, and least lucrative specialty of veterinary medicine. Many young veterinarians envision a "James Herriot" rural lifestyle, but learn in school under the tutelage of instructors like Freeman how difficult and impractical farmwork can be—and choose alternate directions. Tom Hufnagel, however, never wavered from his determination to become a veterinarian and return to the rural life near family and neighbors that he loved.

We are scrunched together in his mobile clinic—a full-size Ford F-250 pickup truck—a specially designed, fully stocked four-wheel veterinary facility, with refrigeration, hot and cold running water, and ultrasound facilities, much fancier than anything Freeman will have available at New Bolton. As he drives

maniacally down a winding, narrow, bumpy, potholed, shoulder-
less, signless road, Tom Hufnagel, a bearded man with a long
ponytail, is talking loudly with his usual rapid-fire delivery.
April, his assistant and loyal friend since high school, nods in
continual affirmation, as Tom remembers how difficult it was to
get started in the veterinary business near the tiny towns of
Harmony and Zelienople, Pennsylvania: how they sat in anxious
vigil during office hours waiting for the phone to ring and wondering if the few scheduled appointments would actually materi-
alize; how Tom and April beat the bushes to persuade farmers
who had traditionally treated animals themselves to trust him
not only in times of crisis, but on a regular preventative basis
because it would benefit their animals and their bank accounts
in the long run.

During the first few years, Hufnagel worked seven days a
week, for he instantly discovered the bane of the veterinarian's
existence, which is the fickleness of his most ardent and seemingly loyal clientele. If clients call with a sick animal and you're
not available, you may not see them again, especially if the
veterinarian they turn to cares for that animal in a satisfactory
manner. Many of his customers are very poor. He's taken trades
in return for his services—work on his cars, livestock, painting,
mowing the grass. Once he accepted a cow that ate eight hundred dollars worth of the shrubs he had planted around his backyard. Another time, he kenneled and treated a cat with multiple
sicknesses for eight months and only charged three hundred and
fifty dollars because that's all the client said they would be willing to pay. Ninety percent of his customers want to know up
front how much it will cost and will tell him in no uncertain
terms their financial limit. Often, the veterinarian decides how
far to go with a given animal based on how much money he is
willing to gamble on his own competence.

Although his most exciting and interesting work may occur in the field, Hufnagel is a rare mixed-practice veterinarian, treating small domestic animals and scheduling regular office hours in equal proportion to the time in which he travels in his mobile clinic.

We turn into a narrow, hilly driveway, pass an attractive ranch house with a customized Dodge Ram Charger and park in front of a rambling, low-slung stable. This is a quarter horse breeder who Tom and April visit twice a week, spring and summer, to help facilitate artificial insemination. We walk into the barn—undoubtedly one of the coldest buildings I have ever been in, even on this mild spring day. Despite the cold, to which he claims to be oblivious ("I never wear socks, winter or summer, snow or ice; I am a very hot-blooded veterinarian"), Hufnagel pulls off his sweatshirt, revealing a black sleeveless T-shirt and a gaudy tattoo of the Aesculapian staff—the veterinary symbol—a winged staff entwined with two serpents. He pulls on a long plastic glove, which reaches from his fingertips over the tattoo to his shoulder, watching while Sandy, the owner, leads the first mare out of its stall, across the barn and into the rack, a rectangular contraption made of steel pipe into which the horse is confined for examination. They begin with the mares they bred last week, checking for ovulation. "By palpating mares a couple of times," he says, "I know how fast they will be growing."

Hufnagel inserts his hand into the mare's rectum, digging out feces by the handful and tossing it into a stainless steel bucket. Slowly, he works his arm inside, buried up to his shoulder. He works quickly, one mare after another; he will examine sixteen mares for Sandy today within the next ninety minutes. Often, he must brace himself with the root pole of the stocks—the pole that prohibits the rear hooves of the horse from kicking him—plant his feet in back of the horse and push. He must push with enough force to overcome resistance from the sphincter muscle, while being careful not to cause a rectal tear. He carries a plastic bottle of lubricant in his back pocket, which he will squirt on his gloved hand from time to time to make entry easier. (When James Herriot made a rectal examination, he needed a bucket of hot water, soap, and a towel. He soaked his arm and gently inserted it into the animal's rectum.) When Hufnagel finishes each exam, he dictates his verdict (Is the horse pregnant? Or when shall she be bred?). Sandy records it in a soiled loose-leaf binder.

After at least a dozen examinations, with Sandy running to answer a phone call, Hufnagel leads me into the back room to show me a strange contraption, an old water heater with a thick foam mattress wrapped around it, held together by what looks like a mile of tattered duct tape. He points to a corral door. "That's where the stud lives. When Sandy's ready to collect semen, she brings in one of the mares to get the stud worked up." When the stud is sufficiently aroused, the mare is returned to her corral and the stud, let loose, embraces the dummy (the water tank with the foam mattress and the duct tape) and mounts it. Sandy then inserts the stud's erect penis into an artificial vagina, collecting semen. She will use this semen to impregnate the mares sent to her for breeding—or she will ship the semen, chilled and incubated in a special container, across the country. I finger the duct tape wound around the foam and water heater contraption. Hufnagel and April laugh, explaining that the horse's hooves come up over the water heater and whip into the mattress with great gusto. Sandy is constantly patching it with duct tape. "Maybe the horse has a duct tape fetish," Hufnagel says.

Tom Hufnagel will charge thirty dollars for this visit, plus five dollars for each palpation and thirty dollars for each ultrasound. He will charge separately for shots or other treatments. April and Sandy list exactly what was done. Sandy will pay on-the-spot for all veterinary services rendered on a daily basis; she will bill her clients individually for services Hufnagel performed.

Back in the truck, Hufnagel once again reminisces about the difficulty of the first few years of practice. "One thing in my favor was that I knew about farming and how to talk a farmer's language. When they say about a cow, 'When was she fresh?,' that means when did she last have a calf? When they say, 'Did she clean?,' that means did she pass the placenta and membrane? If a cow is 'caught,' it means she's pregnant. And if a cow is 'open,' it means she's not pregnant. When a cow is 'coming in,' it means being in heat in ten days and being ready to be bred. When they realize you aren't only a veterinary school vet, they begin to trust you."

His truck says "Hufnagel Veterinary Clinic" and is customized with blue-and-chrome lettering, front and back; the same lettering is in front of his clinic, but initially Hufnagel used a broken-down pickup, which he repaired and equipped with a veterinary cap salvaged at a junkyard. Most of his equipment and furniture were purchased at auctions from retiring veterinarians liquidating their practices. "My mother said that when I was four years old, I was dissecting the innards of the chickens that she was killing on the farm. In high school, the guidance counselor said, 'I understand that you want to be a veterinarian, but getting into veterinary school is so difficult and the road is so long, what is your second choice, what is your alternative?' And I told her point-blank, 'I want to be a veterinarian. There is no second choice or alternative for me.' "

The following day, Hufnagel's young associate, Kenton Rexford, a tall, broad-shouldered, square-jawed veterinarian with a flat-top haircut and an easy smile, studies a thermometer. It reads 106 degrees. The cow's ears are drooping, and she is dehydrated and experiencing difficulty breathing. Suspecting pneumonia, Rexford decides to use intravenous antibiotics, plus a massive injection of fluids. "First I need a bucket. This time a bucket without holes, which is what you gave me the last time."

The farmer, whose name is Bob, is tall, slender, and dirty, as are his son and his father, although perhaps more so than Bob, their cheeks balled up with snuff. As Bob walks across the barn, past three dozen milk cows arranged in three symmetrical rows, he replies: "You said you wanted a bucket last time, not a bucket that holds water."

Rexford rolls his eyes, waiting while April slips a yellow rope around the cow's head, lashing it to the front bars of its stall. April is tall and, like Hufnagel, has a longish nose and long, curly hair that falls down her shoulders and settles inside the collar of her chambray shirt. For eight years, milking cows on the Hufnagel family dairy farm, she waited for Hufnagel to graduate and establish a practice just as he had promised in high school.

Rexford inserts the intravenous needle into a vein in the cow's neck. After an initial struggle, he injects three vials of medication, followed by a bottle of hypertonic saline to increase the cow's blood pressure. Now Kenton Rexford inserts a shiny steel pipe called a speculum into the cow's throat. This will prevent the cow from chewing through the plastic orgastril tube that is passed through the speculum and down to the stomach. Using a device similar to a bicycle pump, he begins pumping fluid from the bucket into the tube. Suddenly the cow pulls away. Its front legs buckle, and she sinks to the ground, all 1,200 pounds of her, with a dull thud. Immediately, she tries to stand back up, front legs clawing at the hay and the dirt, her back legs pushing ineffectively. Her breathing becomes increasingly labored . . . *HaaaHaaaHaaaHaaa* . . . as she struggles desperately, but with quiet resolution, although continuing the struggle, she knows she will not succeed. Looking up at Rexford, Bob says: "Is she lying down on me, or what?" Her head tilts, and then her mouth begins to bubble and foam. Her tongue slips out of the side of her mouth and hangs there, a thick motionless slab.

Though I am probably the last one to realize that the cow is dead, nobody can move; we stand and stare for the longest and most agonizing minute before April, attempting to bring us back to business, says, "Bob?" And after another seemingly endless minute, "Kenton?" For next fifteen minutes, we examine two other milk cows at Bob's farm.

Everyone is grim but trying to smile, pretending, almost politely, that nothing has happened. "But this is the kind of thing you think about late at night," Rexford said later. "No matter how many success stories you tell people, this is the story you will always remember. Most vets want to be perfect. Veterinarians are overachievers in high school. I had nearly a 4.0 average through college. But we can't live with defeat so easily. I'll wake up with this tonight; I won't be able to stop thinking about it. The memory will not go away for a long time, if ever, I'll tell you that right now."

Ed is wearing a short-sleeved plaid shirt. He has a gray-speckled beard and horn-rimmed glasses. He's carrying a spiral notebook and marking down the information given to him by Kenton Rexford. Each cow has a tag with a number on it, and that tag is color-coded.

"The two biggest problems for dairy farmers," says Rexford as he begins a series of seventeen rectal examinations, "are reproduction and—"

"And money," Ed interrupts. "When you are finished with this book about veterinarians, you ought to begin writing a book about the dairy farmer, whose price of milk hasn't gone up in twenty-five years."

"What we're trying to do here," Rexford continues, "is to get the cow pregnant two months after the calf is born. Ideally a cow should have a calf once a year. When they lactate, milk production is best three months after the calf is born, and then the quality of the milk and the rate of production gradually goes down until about the ninth month, when production falls to an unprofitable point, at which time it's time to give the cow a break again, to rest. Not milk her. Of course, at that point also, if we've planned right, the cow is pregnant and about ready to have a calf."

When half of the rectals are done, Rexford takes off his glove and drops it to the ground. "That's about enough for this glove," he says. "But here's a secret of a young veterinarian: Leave the box of gloves on the other side of the barn so that you can walk all the way down to get a new glove, thereby resting your arm." Seventeen rectals are not a lot to give for the average farm veterinarian on any given examination, but it is for a newcomer like Rexford. The manure, which is very wet and slippery, has come up past the cuff of the glove onto his blue coverall and is sticking to his bare arm. He will be encrusted by manure at the end of this day. And it's so cold in this barn that when he pushes through into the anus for the first time, a puff of steam comes out of each cow.

Rexford says, stopping to rest and breathe and moan, "Farmers like to breed their cattle and dairy cows for certain characteristics. Size, being one of them. I wish they would be bred for loose anal tone and lower manure production."

Ed and April laugh.

Periodically, April reaches down and lifts the cuff of the glove up over Rexford's shirt to protect his arms and shoulders from becoming soiled. After each rectal, Rexford shakes the loose manure from his arm into the manure gutter.

In the truck, I ask Rexford how he feels about giving so many rectals in any given day. He doesn't quite know how to answer, although he says that it is an important diagnostic tool, sometimes making the difference between sickness and health, surgery and noninvasive procedures.

"Cows and horses have very strong muscles in their anus and in their gut," he tells me, "stronger than I do in my arm. One of the things you do when you become a food animal veterinarian is try to develop strong fingers and work on your dexterity so that you can move them around when they're immobilized. When I first started working full-time, I'd get tired after about five rectals during the day. And a cow's gut and anus muscles, as well as a horse's, are so strong that they can squeeze your arm and cut off circulation.

"It's very warm inside there," he says, lowering his voice. "It feels kind of soothing and comfortable. An animal's core body temperature is about 100 degrees, and it's very soft and everything is firm and smooth to the touch. But for some students in veterinary school, doing a rectal can actually be very discouraging, especially early on, when they don't know what they're feeling. It's like groping around in a strange room in the pitch dark, looking for a friendly hand—and getting a handful of feces."

Before the next call, we check in at the office, where Tom Hufnagel is seeing patients. Hufnagel is angry at a client he has just seen, a man who refused to accept the notion that his dog had gotten fleas from his house.

"That man sat there, listening to me and nodding as I explained to him how his animal had to have gotten fleas from the place where he lives, which is his home. And I thought logically that if I showed him a flea on his dog . . . so I found a couple of fleas in the animal's coat . . . he'd understand and accept what I'm telling him. So I captured a couple and held them up in front of his face. And I explained he needed to buy flea products to rid his animal of fleas and that he had to vacuum and clean his house. And then he said to his wife, standing up and walking out the door, 'No way. It's impossible. That dog didn't get the fleas in our house.' "

"Remember what James Herriot said?" says Rexford. "People will listen to anyone else but their veterinarian, in terms of what to do with their animal." Rexford's observation reminded me of Herriot's primary nemesis, the local owner of the slaughterhouse, Jeff Mallock, who served as the unofficial animal coroner, whom the farmers often consulted either for diagnosis—or an evaluation of Herriot's treatment. Invariably Mallock's assessment, which usually took place after the animal had died and Mallock had conducted a crude postmortem, involved one of a half-dozen Mallock-derived diseases, including "stagnation of t'lungs, black rot, gastric ulcers or 'golf' stones." Mallock's most frequent and impressive diagnosis (at least to the farmers who sought him out) was "worm in the tail." Had Herriot removed the tail of an ailing cow, according to Mallock, the cow would have surely gotten up and walked away.

Hufnagel listened and nodded impatiently as Rexford talked. But clearly, he wasn't ready to calm down. "I hate it when these situations occur," he said loudly and to no one in particular, and for the rest of the day he seemed unable to shake the memory of his conversation with the disagreeable client. Over and over, at every opportunity, Hufnagel repeated: "When people don't listen to their veterinarians, they are actually mistreating their animals. That angers me, it really does. It puts a knot in my stomach that is impossible to unravel. I'm telling you, I just can't stand it."

# REINDEER WITH A HERNIA

<br>

At the long, battered rectangular table in the commissary of the Pittsburgh Zoo, Steven Marks first explains to his small staff how he hopes to capture one reindeer and anesthetize her. As he outlines the surgical procedure, Karen Lindquist, the certified veterinary technician, compiles a list of equipment and medications to pack into the van. In addition to the obvious surgical paraphernalia, Karen includes extension cords, halogen lamps, spotlights, and heavy rope.

Listening to their discussion, I remind myself how precise their planning must be—and how difficult it is to be precise when doing something for the first time and in an unfamiliar setting. Because of the unpredictable eccentricities of the many species of animals, fish, and birds in a zoo, and because there is not a lot of medical literature to consult, there can be no uniformity of procedure, which is a mainstay in most surgeries for animals or humans alike. No one in this small group, including Marks, and probably few people in the world, has ever removed an umbilical hernia from a North American reindeer, most especially one with an abscess, which undoubtedly caused the hernia—and certainly not in an unlit, unheated stable. But that is the multiple problem and the plan.

At the conclusion of the meeting, Karen disappears down the narrow corridor to the zoo hospital to begin her work, aided by associate veterinarian Don Neiffer. Curator Lee Nesler, a tall, big-boned woman with curly blond hair, fair skin, broad features, and freckled face, suddenly jumps up from the table singing and dancing and making a cacophony of animal noises. But when she sees me in the corner, she blushes. "I forgot you were here," she says.

Steven Marks remains momentarily seated, oblivious to Nesler's commotion, double-checking his list, item by item, before folding his clipboard and gathering his papers. Tall, lanky, and intense, Marks strides purposefully down the connecting corridor, through the hospital, dumping his papers on an old wooden desk in the cluttered office he shares with Neiffer.

Marks has a long, oblong-shaped head. His hair and beard are thick and dark brown, as are his large looping eyebrows. He's wearing a white shirt with a Pittsburgh Zoo iron-on emblem and green pants, a zoo standard. After conversing briefly with Karen and Neiffer, he leaves the building, crosses the parking lot adjacent to the nursery, and hurries into the main exhibit area, calling into his walkie-talkie, a constant companion to all zoo supervisory personnel, to Gus McClung, the zookeeper at the North American hoofed animal exhibit, to open the gate. A tall, soft-spoken man in a soiled baseball cap, Gus had alerted Marks during rounds yesterday morning to "this big sac" hanging down from the stomach of a female reindeer. Marks had leaned over the fence, craning his neck and scrunching his black brows watching intensely as the reindeer cavorted about in the grassy area she called home. In a zoo, careful observation at a respectful distance is the standard way in which animals are preliminarily examined, which in this case was sufficient for Marks to diagnose the hernia. "We're going to have to knock her down," he told Gus, meaning, "we're going to have to put her under anesthesia, examine the area in question, and probably do surgery on it."

At first, Marks had instructed Gus to isolate the reindeer in a stall and to put her on a water-only diet. He had scheduled the procedure two days ahead to allow for all food to be digested. A primary danger in a procedure when anesthesia is necessary is that animals may regurgitate food that they have stored inside of them and suffocate themselves. Or, more commonly, they will regurgitate and then aspirate it into the lungs, which invariably leads to "aspiration pneumonia" within three or four days. This is why Marks will struggle so hard to intubate (insert a breathing tube into the mouth and throat) the animal, so that stomach contents—if brought up—will not go down into the trachea.

But as the day wore on, Marks compulsively returned to study the reindeer in earnest. Even though it was nearly impossible to glimpse her stomach, where the hernia hung in a huge lump, he repeatedly peeked through the hole in the stall door watching as the reindeer paced the tiny, twelve-foot-square stall. Once in a while, he eased himself through the door and stood in the middle of the stall contemplating the skittish creature as she huddled in a corner and eyed him warily. Early that evening, fearing infection, Marks informed Gus, Don, Karen, and Lee that he had decided to schedule surgery for the following day.

When we enter the stable, Gus is hosing down three thick rubber mats on which the procedure will take place. Conferring briefly, Marks and Gus decide to use the ornate oversized hinges on both the stall door leading to the grassy open exhibit area and the door that leads to the main barn or paddock area to lash the reindeer down. The rope will secure the animal during surgery. "Sounds like a plan," Marks says as he snatches his walkie-talkie and returns to the hospital to help Karen with the equipment.

While waiting for Karen and Marks, I ride with Lee Nesler in the Cushman, a tiny three-wheeled mini-truck similar to a golf cart, to pick up raccoon traps, which are set out each night. Raccoons can spread disease to animals, as do pigeons and rats. Each of the three traps set last night have at least one new visitor. Nesler, the curator or chief animal management administrator, holds a cage in her hand, watching the furry predator scurrying back and forth and then hovering in a corner as it begins to contemplate the inevitability of its plight. Nesler talks in a very friendly, soothing manner to the raccoon, as if the raccoon were like all the other creatures in this zoo, a part of the burgeoning community and one of her beloved children. But within the next thirty minutes and probably much sooner, the raccoon will be euthanized.

Getting the reindeer back into the stall area where Gus has laid down the rubber mats (Gus released the animal into a large open-air pen so that he could prepare the stall for the upcoming surgery) is the first problem. Each time Gus separates the reindeer from the herd and pushes her toward the paddock, the reindeer glimpses Neiffer or Marks—and retreats.

Even though it is starting to rain, Marks decides to "knock down" the reindeer outside, in the open. He directs Neiffer to prepare the anesthetic dart similar to a hypodermic needle for the $CO_2$ gun they sometimes use, while he and Gus search the hallway for electrical power. Karen and Nesler carry equipment from the van and arrange it around the stall. The brick stable, originally part of an estate of an early industrialist, is 150 years old. The arched doors are solid steel, the wooden roof is slanted with open beams and tile shingles.

Two long extension cords are required to bring power from Gus's cramped office through the paddock and into the stall. Meanwhile, his air rifle loaded with an anesthetic called ketamine, Neiffer stalks the reindeer up a hill around a grassy knoll and down toward the flat near the stall—unsuccessfully. Neiffer fires. Then he reloads and fires again, missing again. "She's deceptively quick," he says.

Eventually, Neiffer finds the mark, and in a few minutes the reindeer sinks to the ground, groggy and helpless. They carry her into the corral and ease her down on the rubber mats. Marks covers the reindeer's large brown eyes with a blue drape. Nesler busies herself making cooing noises, caressing the reindeer, and picking loose fur and bits of dirt from the reindeer's coat. Meanwhile, Marks is struggling with the intubation. Leaning forward over the reindeer and twisting his hand up her throat, he mumbles, "I just can't . . . get my finger . . . to the epiglottis." And then, in a few minutes, "Finally," he says. "Alright."

Now the reindeer is flipped onto her back. Her front legs are tied together and then lashed with a rope across the stall and to the hinge on the door. Her rear legs are also tied together and lashed to a hinge on the opposite side of the stall. Both ropes are steadied by bales of hay and the rope-pole arrangement that Gus and Marks had originally established. A third bale of hay is used as an instrument table, while a fourth is the base for a toolbox on which sits a halogen light. It shines brightly down on the herniated area. The concrete floor is wet. The mats that Gus put out are also wet and dotted with straw.

Now Karen produces a bucket of warm water. Marks scrubs the furry white abdominal area briskly, twice. Soap suds appear everywhere. Marks takes an electric shaver and shaves the surgical area clean. Neiffer scrubs the area a third time, lifting away loose white and brown hair, and then liberally coats the entire surgical field with Betadine, an orange-brown-colored antiseptic.

Marks puts on a pair of blue coveralls. He empties a cardboard box, turns it upside down, and makes it into a table. Neiffer drapes the table with a sterile cloth. Marks covers the rest of the animal, using four lime green drapes. Karen checks the oxygen and the other equipment for which she will be responsible. Neiffer double-checks her connections and settings. They begin.

The monitor, which has been beating steadily for ten minutes, suddenly records an increased heart rate as Marks cuts into the animal. The yellow ball bouncing on the screen illuminates the corner of the stall, where it has been placed. As Marks cuts and sutures, he wants to know how old the reindeer is. Gus goes into his office to look it up. He returns momentarily to announce that the reindeer is nine.

Now Nesler leans forward and eases herself down on the reindeer, continuing to touch and coo to her, even though the animal is fast asleep. Nesler has big scratches on her legs. She has tied her blond hair into braids so that the strands don't fall into her eyes. Karen regulates the reindeer's breathing, six times a minute, by hand-squeezing a canvas "ambou," or "rebreathing" bag.

The scene is bizarre: instruments on silver trays resting on bales of hay; a yellow-spotlighted area in a darkened, partially abandoned stable; two masked surgeons kneeling on wet ground, cutting, suturing for an hour, and then another hour, not getting up to stretch or joke or drink some water. I can't help thinking of the opening chapter of *All Creatures Great and Small,* in which the young, inexperienced veterinary surgeon James Alfred Wight (Herriot) in Yorkshire Dales in northern England, lies facedown in a pool of icy mud, stripped to the waist, his arm deep inside a straining cow searching vainly for a birthing calf. Almost two hours later, Herriot could be found in the same position, achingly tired, but still fighting to save the calf.

What was different about Herriot's procedure in 1940 and the work being performed in the Pittsburgh Zoo today, of course, is that Marks and Neiffer have technology on their side, at least to a certain extent—and a team of helpers. But in a very real comparative sense, the primitive nature of veterinary medicine, particularly in certain situations, is not very much different from a half-century ago when Herriot began to practice.

Another hour passes. You can hear the birds chirping in the rafters in the stable. You can hear Gus, who quietly and immediately exited because he could not stand the sight of the blood of his animals, shoveling hay and mud and hosing down the paddock area—and singing softly. Plus you hear the constant babble from Lee Nesler's walkie-talkie that is balanced on a cushion and turned up loud.

At some point during that morning, children visiting from an elementary school begin singing "Rudolph the Red Nosed Reindeer" to the remaining members of the herd grazing behind the fence. You wonder how they would respond if they were aware of the intricate and dangerous procedure taking place behind this inconspicuous stall door.

As they work, both Marks and Neiffer become increasingly tense. The flies are buzzing around their heads. They suture with one hand and brush them away with the other. Eventually they begin removing the abscess in the umbilical hernia. Cutting through the animal's skin and digging deep enough to excise the entire area is more difficult than they had expected. Feeling claustrophobic in the dark, eerie, cluttered space, instruments and people clustered all around him, Marks suddenly flings a few pieces of flesh, skin, and swabs to the opposite corner of the room, shouting unintelligibly. This outburst seems to make him feel better. He smiles. Karen looks up at me. "Do you want to feel the softest nose ever invented?"

I kneel down. Karen is right. The reindeer's nose is warm and lightly fuzzy, like well-worn velvet or satin. In fact, it is so soothing in the tense atmosphere, I feel spellbound and remarkably peaceful. The scene swirls around me: Marks with his thick beard and dark hair, kneeling down beside this cuddly creature, eradicating a dangerous infection, preserving its life; hay piled up all around and enclosing and enhancing our special intimacy; Gus singing spirituals, which echoes through the corridors of the ancient building; and Nesler, pressing her warm body down against this tiny reindeer, meticulously cleaning her coat and cooing quietly—calming and fortifying one of God's most helpless creatures. This is a moment and a snapshot I will never forget.

# AQUAZOO

When I arrive at the hospital the morning after the reindeer procedure, Marks and Karen are on their way to examine a loggerhead green sea turtle that, some months ago, had developed lesions on its shell. Suspecting a cancerous tumor, Marks had biopsied the shell, but the results were inconclusive, meaning, said Marks, "We weren't able to learn anything from it—not that the results weren't saying anything. After all, how many green sea turtles do we biopsy in a given decade?"

This is a message that is communicated repeatedly by Marks, Neiffer, and other veterinarians who deal with "exotic" animals. An inordinate amount of medical research has been conducted on animals, but most of it for the benefit of humans. Animals cured or healed through modern medical technology will usually be domestic or of the food animal variety—dogs, cats, cows, and pigs—for which a track record of care and treatment exists. The ancestors of most zoo animals either healed themselves or died in the wilds. At zoos, veterinarians have just started introducing modern medical techniques to the exotic animal world. In fact, the Pittsburgh Zoo, one of the largest in the United States, and not unlike most other zoos, added veterinarians to its full-time staff less than a decade ago. Despite lack of a definitive diagnosis, Marks and Neiffer aggressively and persistently treated the sea turtle from the beginning. In this case, the results have been quite positive.

At the Aquazoo, a separate building on the complex, a zookeeper climbs on top of a tank the circumference of a large hot tub, perhaps about nine feet deep, balances himself on his stomach, and attempts to attract the turtle's attention. Turtles are known to be slow. The tortoise and the hare story is one we all remember. But in the water, they become deceptively fast, dodging the zookeeper's extended arms and Marks's net like a running back avoiding an oncoming tackler. It takes the keeper and Marks about fifteen minutes to grab the turtle, lift it out of the tank, and lower it to the ground. We attract a crowd immediately—kids who want to see what the zoo doctor is doing and get a close-up of the gigantic turtle. Marks had planned to conduct a quick examination and apply the treatment to the turtle on the floor out in the open. But now he and the keeper hurriedly carry the turtle through an emergency exit and into the bowels of the exhibit building.

Over the past month, Marks and Neiffer have been scraping the infected area regularly with Betadine while applying a triple antibiotic/antifungal combination treatment, covered with a Tegaderm patch, a thin, translucent silicone membrane, held firm with a thick coating of epoxy paste. The lesions gradually filled in—re-epithelized—eliminating the portal of entry for the infection. Because so many procedures at this and other zoos are being attempted for the first time ever, much of what veterinarians are required or forced to do are makeshift—like turning the stable into an operating room, or making this little concrete-floored passageway into an examination room, and using epoxy paste to protect a wound.

Zoo veterinarians are a new and relatively small, tight-knit group in the veterinary community. The first full-time zoo veterinarian in the world, Dr. Charles Spooner, was appointed to the London Zoo in 1829, while American zoos waited until the turn of the century for Dr. H. Amling, Jr., to be hired away from a traveling circus by the Bronx Zoo in New York. There are not a great many full-time zoo positions in the United States today, although with the advent of theme parks and Sea World–like facilities, the job market for experts in wild animals is growing steadily.

Now Karen strings her ever-present extension cord from a nearby outlet and connects it to a hair drier so that the Tegaderm-epoxy treatment can be dried quickly. I notice the turtle's awkward-looking front and hind flippers as he sits there with the zookeeper holding them down. No wonder they're so slow on dry land. The zookeeper tells me that turtles are kind of dangerous. Often, if he's not careful, the turtle scratches him when he lifts him up out of the water.

The keeper, Karen, and Steven Marks gather around the turtle and wait for the epoxy to dry. Karen pulls up a bucket to sit on. But Marks kneels down on one knee. I'm amazed at how long he can remain in that position. In describing the qualities of a good veterinarian, many experts refer to a superior athletic ability; indeed, most veterinarians, especially wildlife or farm vets, are trim and fit. I can't remember running into a veterinarian who is excessively overweight or out of shape. Courage is another qualification that all veterinarians must possess. A veterinarian's work combines the skills of a mountain climber, a law enforcement officer, and a family practice physician. I remember how Marks and Neiffer staggered and creaked to their feet after the reindeer procedure, like two of the oldest men alive, and how they forced themselves to place one foot ahead of the other, walking. It was incredibly painful to be down, squatting, without knee pads, for that long. "My knees hurt for weeks afterwards," Neiffer recalled.

The Aquazoo is dark and dramatic from the spectator's point of view, hundreds of exotic fishes in lush, dimly lit aquariums, but amazingly drab and ordinary on the other side, in the bowels of the exhibit area. Everything inside is bare. Bare wood. Bare plastic pipe. Concrete. Everything is jerry-rigged and utilitarian. Tubes. Plywood. Water. Stains. Wires. Step ladders. Wire clothes hangers, unfurled. Strings. Old yellowed patches of masking tape. There are many exotic and unpleasant aromas. Even the turtle smells rank and putrid.

When the turtle is happily back at home in the water, we visit a penguin with bandaged feet. The rocks in the exhibit, actually constructed of plaster and papier-mâché, are hard on the bottoms of penguins' feet and often cause chafing and infection. A redesign of the exhibit will include foam-padded flooring. There are seventeen penguins to care for in this exhibit, all with black and white feathers, almost like formal wear, spruced up with nifty, long, fringelike yellow feathers around the neck and head. Most of these penguins, which range in size from king penguins, about forty inches tall and thirty to forty pounds, to rockhoppers, twelve inches tall and three to five pounds, were wild-caught on islands off the coast of Chile. "Most people think penguins are from the Antarctica, but the majority live on the southern tip of Africa and the southern tip of New Zealand—close to Antarctica but not on it. There are a number of birds who go to Antarctica—flying birds who visit and depart—but not the penguin."

A common problem of penguins in captivity is pododerma-titis, more commonly known as "bumble foot." Many factors come into play causing bumble foot, including the fact that penguins become dirtier in zoos than in the wilds because they are often forced to stand in excrement for long periods of time. Also, upward pressure from the flat-surfaced floor is unending, causing open irritation and abrasions. Bacteria eventually seeps into such wounds, causing abscesses, ulcers, lameness. More modern zoos or those with more resources like Sea World actually include snow in the penguin exhibits, minimizing cases of bumble foot. In the wilds, most of the heaviest penguins are usually living on snow, a soft, nonabrasive surface. "Pododerma-titis," said Marks, "is a predictable problem of captivity."

Marks and Neiffer unrelentingly treated the penguin over a period of two months, until it became clear that the bird was irreversibly harmed, necessitating euthanization. "It is very unrewarding to treat bumble foot," Neiffer said.

We join the Aquazoo curator, Randy, and two zookeepers for a routine physical on Chuckles the dolphin. Chuckles is a very unique animal—the only Amazon River dolphin in captivity in the United States. Chuckles was one of a dozen Amazon River dolphins that were brought here in the 1960s. But he's now the only remaining survivor and a threatened species, soon to be endangered, Marks speculates. "The rivers are the first avenues for development in third world countries. They'll be dammed up, cutting off food sources for fish and wildlife. And then all of the animals in the rivers will be gone. The natives in the Congo consider dolphins sacred, and they don't touch them; it's the people who come in and disrupt the area. The rivers are the first to go. They don't have roads in the Amazon; you travel by boat."

Marks, who grew up in Quakertown, near Philadelphia, was a marine biology major at the Florida Institute of Technology until he realized that his role model, Jacques Cousteau, was atypical of the life he might eventually lead. He quickly altered his goal to something more practical: veterinary medicine. While earning his undergraduate degree in microbiology, Marks worked evenings as a volunteer at the University of Florida School of Veterinary Medicine shoveling out stalls and helping with treatments. "I worked in a swine unit one summer. It would be 100 degrees outside and I'd be inside the barn, using a steam-jenny; I lost a lot of weight. I also worked for a large-animal veterinarian, and then on a wildlife conservation plantation and everywhere else I could to gain experience. Grades are important in getting into veterinary school, but experience is most important. I tend to prosper in that kind of environment; I was fortunate enough to get in on my first try."

Marks remembers sitting with classmates, adorned in cap and gown, on the day of his graduation from veterinary school, thinking to himself, "Now what?" From high school onward, his goals had evolved—from gaining acceptance into veterinary school to this moment, graduation—an eight-year quest now suddenly achieved. He cannot remember who gave the keynote address, but the simple insight of the speaker's message struck an integral chord—that veterinarians should become more involved in conservation issues. "We deal with animals, we're scientists, and we possess a unique appreciation for wildlife; veterinarians are in a key position to make an impact." That is when Marks resolved to attempt the nearly impossible and become a wildlife veterinarian—one of the most exclusive and elite specialties in the profession. The speaker concluded his remarks with a quote from Albert Schweitzer: "It is man's sympathy with all creatures which makes him truly a man."

Marks took a job in his hometown of Quakertown, Pennsylvania, in a mixed practice (large and small animals), where he could gain experience with a wide array of animals. Another option was to do a wildlife residency, but that meant burdening his parents for support, increasing the amount of his already substantial loans, and returning to school for at least two more years; it was too much. The Quakertown practice was large, with four veterinarians on the road and four more in-house at the clinic, a laboratory—a total of thirty-two employees.

Marks began seeing dairy and equine clients mostly, and joined the rotation for emergency duty, carrying a pager day and night. It seemed to be detonating on his belt constantly. "When you're on duty, and the pager starts going off, and you've just finished dinner and you're trying to relax, your blood pressure goes sky high. And then you get home from an emergency, it's midnight, you're just falling asleep and the pager goes off again, and it's a cow in dystocia, so you spend the rest of the early morning hours dealing with the cow, and then another page—a cow needs a C-section or a horse with a colic. And none of the owners appreciate the fact that you are up at three A.M., I guess because they're up with you or they're paying for your services." Marks loved many aspects of his first job, being out of doors, on farms—the rural environment was appealing—but he hadn't forgotten the notion of conservation or the Schweitzer quote that inspired him.

During the year at Quakertown, he forged a professional relationship with the owner of a small traveling circus with elephants, camels, zebras, and a few other exotics. Plus, there were a number of clients in the area with exotic birds; none of the other veterinarians on staff expressed much interest or expertise. There were actually two specific and closely related specialties that interested him—zoo medicine and wildlife medicine. But wildlife medicine, which deals with wild animal herds and animal population medicine, was less practical at this point in his life. Experience gained during an externship in his senior year at the Miami Metro Zoo had been instrumental in his ability to care for a variety of species. The University of Florida had had two board-certified wildlife veterinarians on staff, who had helped shape Marks's ideas and provide key experiences. "What I've done in life as long as I can remember," Marks said, "is to trust myself enough to follow my interests, which is what I did in veterinary school and in Quakertown."

The pleasure and the challenge—the aspect that makes veterinary medicine so special—is the continued opportunity to learn. "You've got every species in the world to work with, and every possible disease that could effect each species, in every facet or specialty of medicine. An MD is dealing with one species and one facet of medicine, whether it be ophthalmology or gastroenterology or whatever. It's very specific." He discovered that diversity led to knowledge and a plethora of rich experience, which he parlayed into his own private practice in Exton, Pennsylvania, closer to Philadelphia. In addition to doing farm animal work and maintaining his other professional relationships, he was asked to develop a preventive medicine program for the animals at the Elwood Park Zoo. Following his interests, as usual, he volunteered his free time to expand this tiny zoo's facilities. "I was out there with a jackhammer breaking the asphalt trying to lay lines to help bring in water to a veterinary exam area. I spent a lot of my free time at the zoo, helping them do different things that needed to be done."

A unique aspect of veterinary medicine, not so easily achievable in other professions, is the opportunity for young veterinarians to forge their own destinies. Entrepreneurship is appreciated; self-starters are encouraged and rewarded. Marks accompanied the director of the Elwood Park Zoo to the annual meeting of the American Zoo and Aquarium Association, today called American Zoological Association, where he learned that the veterinarian position at the Pittsburgh Zoo was vacant. "It was a one in a million shot, but it worked; I got the job."

Amazon River dolphins are more difficult to care for than the more common marine dolphin, Marks says. They require higher temperatures and shallower water facilities—and have more complicated diets. A big problem in caring for these animals is tank sterility. It is easier for bacteria and fungus to grow in fresh water than in submarine water, and it is easier to keep a submarine system sterile. "Today we have the knowledge and the technology to care for these dolphins—we would not lose them—but they are no longer easy to get."

Randy the curator grabs Chuckles by the snout, holds his teeth together, and pulls him onto the canvas stretcher designed with sheepskin on one side so that the animal is not harmed. There are holes in the stretcher for flippers to be inserted, plus an opening at the end of the stretcher for venting, just in case a semen or fecal sample is necessary. This also provides access to the genitalia and rectum. Chuckles wears that prototypical contented Charlie Brown dolphin smirk, as if everything he sees amuses him and that he is pretty much above it all. A Velcro strap is wrapped around his mouth to prevent biting. Two eight-foot planks are extended across the railings of the exhibit. A scale and a chain are hung on these boards, and there's a hook on the end. The stretcher with Chuckles inside is hung on the hook, and his weight in kilos is recorded.

Meanwhile, Marks is attempting to draw blood for a complete blood count (CBC) differential and chemical screen from the soft tissue in the flippers, similar to the tissue space on a human hand between the fingers. Periodically somebody will bend down and pour water on Chuckles to be certain he doesn't overheat. Generally, the marine dolphin is easy to bleed. "You see veins everywhere." But the Amazon River dolphin can be much more difficult because their venous arterial systems are not as obvious, and the tail fluke, which is the best place to get blood from a marine dolphin, is not a good site in the Amazon River variety.

Thus the challenge in getting blood from a dolphin, Marks says, is that you can't see the vein. "It's called a 'blind stick,' meaning you have to know the anatomy of the animal carefully enough so that you can imagine or sense where the veins are."

Tasks that are basically routine in human hospitals, such as drawing blood for diagnostic tests and procedures, are significant challenges in a zoo atmosphere, requiring years of experience and rare expertise. Blood is drawn twice a week from veins in the ear of elephants, for example. Perhaps most difficult to locate is the vein of a snake. As the physical examination continues, Chuckles's teeth are cleaned and cultures are taken from his blowhole. He is scrubbed down with Betadine and coated with an antifungal agent before being returned to the water.

Chuckles's physical going smoothly, Marks leaves Karen, Don Neiffer, Randy, and the rest of the crew while he continues his morning rounds. I join him. On our way, we run into Lisa, who was once a volunteer dolphin trainer. In fact, she shows us her hand, which is scarred up pretty badly. She had been hurt by Chuckles, who yanked her into the water. "Oh, he only wanted to take a swim," Lisa said defensively. But later, Marks informed me that Chuckles had been getting rough with the entire staff and they have now gone to a hands-off training policy, a system of poles with balls on the end called "target training." This isn't particularly what the dolphins appreciate, and their training has perhaps suffered, "but having Lisa pulled into the water like that, and hurt, was a sobering experience for the zoo staff," Marks said.

# PRIMATES—AND
# OTHER WARRIORS

· ———————————————————— ·

I s there a primate war going on?" I asked Steven Marks one
day on rounds, as we walked toward the tropical forest exhibit. I had overheard a couple of keepers discussing tension and
aggression in the primate exhibit over the past few days.

"More like a lemur war," he tells me. "Two days ago, I had to
sew up a piece of a lemur's ear."

"Why are they battling?"

Marks shrugged and rolled his eyes. "Interspecies aggression is
a big problem for primates, especially in captivity. But who
knows why, specifically? A bongo killed a zebra not too long ago,
but no one will know what happened until bongos or zebras start
to talk." We are now on our way to examine two tree kangaroos
who have been fighting. A keeper has told Marks that one of the
animals has been slightly injured.

Walking through the Primate Center, Marks describes the

challenge of an intraspecies environment. We see monkeys from different species grooming one another, which pleases him, but he is frustrated by conditions of artificiality. The paint and fiberglass from the trees and rocks, for example, have been chipped away by monkeys constantly ripping at them with their hands and chewing on them, and the residue causes a rash in some monkeys—a contact dermatitis—which he and Neiffer are forever treating. The tree trunks are made of steel tubes covered by concrete and fiberglass. He disapproves of how the chains have been looped together on a swing for the woolly monkeys. He's afraid that the monkeys, jumping from bar to bar and swing to swing, will entangle arms or legs in the loops of the chain. He makes a note to discuss this problem with a keeper.

At the gorilla cages, Marks warns me not to look the animals directly in the eye. "Gorillas get nervous when you look them square in the eye." I have no interest in looking a gorilla square in the eye; they are big, hostile, and imposing, and I don't want them to look back at me. One female gorilla in the collection had been living with one male for ten years and never got pregnant. Finally they were separated and a new male was put in with her, and she got pregnant immediately, "which tells you something about gorillas and reinforces what we already knew about human beings," Marks says.

At the tree kangaroo exhibit, a male kangaroo, a fuzzy, lumpy, goofy-looking creature with a thick, heavy tail, has been trying to seduce a female with a shimmering red-brown coat—a hostile process that has prompted the keeper's call. "The male is ready," the zookeeper says, "but the female isn't—and so the male is hurting her." They are sitting there, staring at each other when we arrive, breathing hard, as if they were just finishing a battle. The zookeeper says that the female kangaroo has been teasing the male kangaroo, leading him along, allowing him to approach her and then suddenly fighting back.

"The wound is superficial," says Marks, after studying it through the glass of the exhibit, "but it looks raw and painful. We'll keep an eye on it, but I don't think it requires my intervention right now."

Before leaving that day, we stopped in to see the reindeer on which Marks and Neiffer had operated a few days ago. She was up and about, walking around. Gus tells Steve: "During the surgery, I was praying for the reindeer and I was praying for you. God did not want that little animal dead; you were the blessed angel sent to save it."

The following Saturday begins a long weekend off for Marks. I meet with Don Neiffer, who has just talked with a zookeeper who reported a problem with one of the gorillas, Mary. She suspects there might have been a fight and that Mary might have been hurt.

It is difficult for Neiffer to observe Mary or make any sort of preliminary diagnosis from the exhibit area—a classic problem for the zoo or wildlife vet. For an unfettered view, we climb three stories up to the flat roof of an adjoining building. Even from here and with the aid of high-powered binoculars, he cannot get a clear view of Mary's leg; the gorilla has ensconced herself with her offspring surrounding and protecting her. The keeper calls her partner with her walkie-talkie. "Grab the party mix out of the cooler and come up to the roof."

In a few minutes, armed with a large plastic bag of goodies, the keeper tosses handfuls of Fig Newtons, raisins, peanuts, and pretzels down at the gorillas, who are delighted by the sudden treats raining down on them from the sky. Mary, unfortunately, remains oblivious to the activity. Neiffer admits that something does seem to be wrong, but it is impossible to know unless he can see her move around or glimpse the leg in close quarters.

"Maybe she's acting weird because she's pregnant," he says hopefully, wagging his brows in anticipation. Rare animals giving birth in a zoo are major and important events—and are sometimes unanticipated by the zoo doctors. Because animals have the tendency to mask all weaknesses and protect themselves and their offspring, they will try to conceal pregnancies, as well as injuries. And because animals are basically large, lumpy creatures and veterinarians do not look at them carefully on a daily basis, it is not out of the question for a veterinarian to come to work one morning and discover an animal nursing an infant—or a half-dozen infants—and be taken by surprise. Keepers maintain a constant awareness of the mounting activities of the animals in their charge, and usually the veterinarians know the animals are pregnant, although predicting with great accuracy the day or week of birth is often a problem. Two giraffes were born in November; Marks and Neiffer had predicted late December. Earlier that year, porcupines were born, as was a bison—events that took the entire zoo staff by surprise.

Before climbing down from the roof, the keeper says, "Wait, I want to show you something." She leads us to a tiny dormer with a trapdoor that she unlocks and swings open, revealing a peephole down into the exhibit area below where the orangutans are located. As I peer down into the glass-enclosed area, I notice that it is soundproof. It had never occurred to me, but the animals cannot hear the people who come to watch them. It makes sense. They are not distracted or frightened by excited children and agitated parents; inside the exhibit it is more peaceful than their natural habitat and the climate is controlled for comfort. In the wilds, orangutans live thirty-sixty feet high in the tropical forest canopy, which is how the exhibit is arranged—in a vertical design, taller than it is deep.

Looking up and spotting us spying on them, the orangs grip the wires of the cyclone fence bordering the exhibit and start to climb up to greet us. "Look at those hands," the keeper croons. "Aren't they absolutely beautiful?"

"Better watch out," Neiffer says, pointing at the orangutan leading the upward climb. "That guy is puckering his lips . . ."

"Yeah, he's spit in my face more times than I can count," the keeper says, "but he sure is cute, just the same."

A major surprise for veterinarians and other animal management personnel is the way in which the animals they treat and sometimes cure relate to them. Making rounds with Marks one day, we stop to examine a natural habitat exhibit of the leopard, which creeps warily toward the cyclone fence where Marks is standing, opens its mouth, bares its teeth, and hisses. A boy who has been watching the interaction between animal and doctor asks if the leopard is hungry.

"No," said Marks, "not hungry; just wary. He doesn't like the guy who carries the blow dart or air rifle." Sooner or later, if they remain in Pittsburgh or any other major zoo long enough, every animal will probably be knocked down, if not because of disease, wound, or infection, then as part of a zoo's normal health maintenance program. Usually, animals typecast human beings by smell; the odors of medicines veterinarians use on their patients are distinctive and reminiscent of the pain they once endured. Kathy, the zookeeper who works with lions and tigers, told me: "All the cats really know Steve and Don, and they don't like them. I try to avoid going into the same room when a painful procedure is going on and while the animal is conscious because I don't want the cats to associate me with the vets."

As Marks approaches the exhibit to examine an elephant he

had recently treated for edema, the animal looked up and then gradually retreated. "Oh, he sees you," the zookeeper smiled.

"He likes me," Marks laughs.

"I don't think so," the keeper replies.

The elephants are being hosed down by the keeper when we arrive. The zookeeper is incredibly skillful in guiding the elephant with a stick. She pokes the elephant in one part of the body and the elephant responds by sinking down on one knee. She lifts the elephant's ears and squirts behind his head. Guided by the stick, the elephant subsequently drops down on two legs and rolls over on its back, allowing the keeper to squirt the elephant's body from head to foot. But elephants are the most dangerous animals in the zoo. "They kill more keepers than lions, tigers, leopards, and bears combined," Marks says. "The American Zookeepers Association is considering a hands-off policy for keepers of elephants, modifying how elephants are trained, because of how dangerous they are."

I ask if they are dangerous because they are dumb or if, because of their size, they bumble around and inadvertently hurt people.

"Elephants are not dangerous because they are stupid; they are dangerous because they are very smart and calculating. They view people as part of the overall hierarchy of their life, just as they do other male and female animals of all species. And if they feel threatened, they won't hesitate to attack. You can almost predict when elephants turn on a keeper. The elephant will be flaring its ears and acting different toward that particular keeper, but they will not do anything blatant—until the opportunity presents itself. A woman keeper stumbled over a log in an exhibit recently and then suddenly, during that second of vulnerability, the elephant turned and attempted to head press her into the ground. It is well thought out, almost like a planned murder." Elephants will also throw things. Marks knew an elephant who would pick up rocks and hurl them at a tourist train. "Elephants," says Marks, "are incredibly accurate bombardiers." He shakes his head as we walk. "These animals. They're great. You get comfortable working on them. You touch them and play with them and talk to them. But you better be careful."

Marks is not so careful at the tiger exhibit, however. This exhibit is especially well designed, with thick foliage, a waterfall, and a deep pool in which the tigers can swim. Marks calls this design "landscape immersion architecture," meaning, "immersing the animal in its natural habitat so that the public can see how it really lives; you conceal as best you can the bars and fences which surround the area. This also works out well for the animal because it makes him feel so much more at home." Marks motions toward a Siberian tiger watching us and says, "Let's go look at this animal. He's so beautiful."

Recognizing his doctor, the tiger stands directly in front of us, leaning his large front paws on the cyclone fence. He is nearly as tall on four legs as I am on two. Instinctively, Marks pokes his fingers through the fence and strokes the tiger's nose, a gesture the tiger answered momentarily with a contented snuffle. This very intimate moment is one of the special rewards of a profession that is not particularly well respected or subsidized. Perhaps because of this special intimacy Marks lingers a moment too long. Suddenly, Kathy, the zookeeper, who has been observing the scene from the background, screams: "Steve! Steve! Watch! Watch!"

First I hear a strong hissing sound. Then Marks jumps. "Oh my God! He got me!" Marks begins to run in circles and shake himself, jumping up and down. "He nailed me!" Marks screams. The tiger was marking its territory. "He nailed me with spray," Marks repeats. "Urine. There are few things in the world that smell worse than tiger piss," Marks says as we quickly retreat back to the zoo hospital washroom. "This is the first time I ever got nailed in the face, but it's probably the best place to get it. Once you get tiger piss in your clothes, you never get it out."

Zoo nutrition is becoming an increasingly important and challenging aspect of a veterinarian's job. In Pittsburgh, there are five thousand animals to feed daily. Each meal for each species must be designed to accommodate age, sex, size, pregnancy, and exercise levels, plus nutritional and calorie requirements. Food must also be appealing to the taste and tradition of the animal being fed. A weekly zoo grocery list may include one thousand pounds of fruits and vegetables for animals such as giraffes and elephants, six hundred pounds of seafood for birds and AquaZoo residents, fifteen hundred crickets and mealworms to be fed to reptiles, twenty-five hundred pounds of grain products and four thousand pounds of hay for hoofed animals like zebras and elks, plus seven hundred pounds of meat for lions, leopards, and tigers, not to mention high- and low-protein biscuits, primarily for monkeys.

Marks and Neiffer learn about taste preference from the zookeepers who note which food items are rejected by animals and which are gobbled up. Some animals have palettes so sensitive that they will eat only items from their native area; for example, certain species of eucalyptus must be cultivated or imported for the zoo's koalas.

"In the zoo field," says Lee Nesler, "veterinarians are like detectives." By this Nesler means that veterinarians, unlike most other animal or human doctors, don't often enjoy the luxury of intense on-the-scene examination. Veterinarians most often diagnose and prescribe based upon information gathered through an animal's history, through personal observation, and through interviews of other observers, primarily keepers and curators.

Marks or Neiffer "round" through the zoo regularly, however, looking for anything abnormal, from odd eye expressions to weight loss to untoward patterns of behavior.

One very interesting detective case the veterinarians were currently solving involved the reason a howler monkey fractured its arm. As Don Neiffer set the monkey's tiny, brown arm in a cast, he referred to it as a "nutritional problem." In kids, this would be called rickets. Nutritional problems endanger the whole troop of howlers, especially the young.

Back in his cluttered office, Neiffer consults his computer. Showing a printout of the howlers' daily diet, he then explains the limitations and difficulties in feeding animals in a zoo. "We would like to think that monkeys eat what we give them, but there are factors of individual preference that come into play, as well as the process of socialization. That is, a certain animal may be on the bottom of the barrel of the social hierarchy, like this young howler, and consequently not be allowed to eat some of the things they really want or need to eat to stay healthy." They also choose food preferentially. Some animals don't like biscuits, while others have no interest in fruit. And some animals, like people, have much more active metabolisms.

Steven Marks actually discovered the answer to the howler monkey nutritional problem by noticing a sore on the monkey's mouth that is usually related to a lack of vitamin D. Further observation of the howler's feeding patterns proved his thesis. The howler was preferentially eating the fruit out of the feed, thus ignoring the well-balanced primate biscuits, which contain most of the vitamins required for good health. These primate biscuits are designed to meet the nutritional requirements of the macaque, which is the traditional laboratory monkey. No one really knows the nutritional requirements of any specific monkey except for the macaque monkey, which in fact are very different from howlers and other primates.

"In the wilds, they spend 90 percent of their time browsing. Feeding is a primary behavioral stimulus. They peel, poke, eat. A biscuit certainly does not enrich any part of their behavior. We really don't know much about the nutritional requirements about our collection. No one has ever done a study. Here we have orangutans that are fat and gorillas that are skinny, and we feed them the same thing. It's a mystery and a challenge."

Later, at an animal management meeting, when curators and veterinarians meet with zoo administrators, Steven Marks complained bitterly about a new fountain recently installed at the zoo. Someone had inaugurated the fountain by throwing pennies into it—"to get people to throw money in." Marks remembers reading about a harbor seal in the San Diego Zoo whose stomach yielded $2.57 in pennies, nickels, and dimes sucked up from the bottom of a fountain; the seal eventually died of copper toxicity. "So if we're worried about copper toxicity and the health and safety of animals, don't put coins in the water. We don't need the money that bad."

# TUSKECTOMY

Zoo animals aren't like cars or houses. Because they are mostly endangered, they cannot easily be replaced. So when the tusk (tooth) of a ten-year-old elephant became infected, Marks and Neiffer became increasingly concerned. After unsuccessfully treating it on their own for many months, they began to worry that the infection would track up into the brain and cause neurological damage that would eventually kill the animal. Thus they began to plan a tusk extraction, more commonly referred to at the zoo as a "tuskectomy."

Marks and Neiffer had never participated in a tusk extraction, and so they began to reach out to veterinary centers throughout the United States to build a competent tuskectomy team to perform the procedure: Twenty veterinarians from the United States, including a dentist from the University of Florida's dental school, Boyd Welch, who had conducted, worldwide, dozens of tuskectomies, were invited to Pittsburgh to be part of this highly unusual event.

In almost all veterinary procedures, including the tuskectomy, "the knockdown," the process of sedating and putting the animal to sleep in order to connect it to the anesthesia machine, is very challenging—and dangerous. It is almost impossible to weigh most zoo animals, which is how dosage is calibrated, so it is difficult to know exactly how much sedative to dole out. Veterinarians have no choice but to guess and confront the obvious pitfalls. Overmedicate and an animal might never wake up. Undermedicate and you risk having a half-sedated animal stumbling around, fracturing a leg or injuring itself in other ways. Undermedication may also seriously endanger zoo personnel.

Veterinary medicine is also the only profession in the world, aside from the hunters in a few primitive outback areas in New Guinea, Borneo, or Peru, whose most critical tool of the trade is a blowpipe. Loaded with pressurized pneumatic syringe darts, connected to hypodermic needles that are designed to inject at the point of contact, the blowpipe, varying in length from four to eight feet, initiates the knockdown. $CO_2$-powered air rifles are also employed for the knockdown, but the noise often frightens the animal and sounds a warning of impending trouble. Blowpipes are often the method of choice in cold weather when the $CO_2$ seems less effective or for shorter procedures when a dart might be removed more easily. For larger animals, such as grizzly bears, many zoo veterinarians will use what is called a "Cap-Chur" rifle, which employs darts with a .22 caliber powder charge, along with the $CO_2$ delivery system. The "Cap-Chur" rifle has lost its popularity because of the tissue trauma it causes, now avoidable with the development and sophistication of the pressurized darts.

Knocking down an elephant posed one additional and potentially dangerous complication: Because it weighed so much, the elephant could actually be injured or killed simply by crashing to the ground. An animal that falls backward after rearing up during an injection can fracture its skull; an animal that falls forward may puncture an eye. But the elephant knockdown at the Pittsburgh Zoo that day was perfectly choreographed by three veterinary anesthesiologists from Ohio State University who studied the elephant so carefully and infused the drugs so precisely and directed their crew of helpers and technicians with such crisp efficiency that the operation was flawlessly performed.

A moment after the injection, the elephant's eyes fogged over. Her legs became rubbery. And then, the masterful finishing touch: As the elephant began to collapse, the support crew went into action, maneuvering with instinctive precision, so that the elephant thudded down fast asleep and injury-free—on a perfectly positioned queen-sized Serta Perfect Sleeper mattress.

Later, I discovered that the elephant had actually been partially acclimated to the procedure by the keepers so that she would be ready for this day—and not be surprised by the heavy straps that she would have to wear around her waist. The straps were essential, since there was a very real possibility that the elephant would be unable to stand after the procedure and might need to be lifted to her feet. In fact, while all of this work was taking place inside the elephant complex, the labor crew was erecting an emergency scaffolding to be positioned over the elephant and connected to a four-ton hoist. Inflatable mattresses used in disaster situations to lift tractor trailers with heavy loads were also at the ready. "If the elephant is not standing by the end of the day," said Marks, "it probably won't ever get up."

The next phase was also dramatic, very labor-intensive and quite ingenious. The elephant was chained in place to spikes embedded into the concrete. Truck tire inner tubes were inflated and placed between the sleeping elephant's legs and under other soft and delicate areas to avoid inflammation and breathing or neuromuscular difficulties—or facial nerve paralysis. Ointment was applied to the eyes to protect the cornea from drying out. A tire was placed on the right side of the elephant's head with the eye in the hole expressly to protect the eye from harm.

With the elephant down, a pulse oximeter, which measures oxygen saturation of arterial blood, is attached to the vulva. Marks and Neiffer put on plastic shoulder-length sleeves and gloves to insert rectal probes for an accurate internal temperature reading. In ordinary surgical procedures, an EKG monitor is attached with alligator clips directly to an animal, but for the elephant the clips are attached to metal hypodermic needles inserted through the skin. More probes for medication supplementation are inserted into the elephant's ears, which are thick, like heavy flaps of rubber.

Although most animals receive many different drugs during a knockdown, including ketamine and Valium, an especially potent agent, called carfentanil citrate, an opiate ten thousand times more powerful than morphine, was administered to the elephant. Using carfentanil citrate, gloves and masks are a must for the entire surgical staff—"a drop on a human membrane will kill you," Neiffer said. A "crash cart" with reversal agents, ambou bags, and a CPR board is also mandatory for possible emergencies.

Intubation was exceedingly difficult. A veterinarian from Cornell University explained in a grunting, sweating monologue, his bare arm and shirtless shoulder buried deep in the elephant's throat, as he searched for the open airway. "It is very tight in here and the tightness causes your arm to swell; when it swells, you lose your sensation and you have an increasingly difficult time trying to successfully complete the intubation—and then remove your arm from the elephant's mouth."

But the primary equipment necessary for the actual procedure surprised me. I had expected "low tech," but for certain parts of the procedure the veterinarians worked with almost "no tech." A variable-speed reversible drill with an inch-thick drill bit and a foot-long extender was used to dig deep into the root of the pulp cavity of the tusk. A steel mallet was employed to hammer large chisel-shaped spikes around the tusk to disengage it from the stump. Then came the coup de grâce, right at the point when the tusk was about to be extracted:

"Okay," said Boyd Welch, a man whom some of the helpers referred to as Dr. Tuskectomy. He was a slightly paunchy, rumpled man who might have passed for an overaged bouncer. After lying on a cold concrete floor for half an hour, showered with bloody abscessed bone pulp and tooth and blood particles, he resembled a laborer in a Chicago meatpacking house. "Okay," he repeated. "Give me that pipe wrench!" In an instant, with a quick flick of his bloody wrist, Dr. Tuskectomy yanked the tusk out. Everyone in that room, except for the sleeping elephant, winced with pain.

There was considerably more work to do, cleaning up the infection and disconnecting the probes and tubes, but within an hour of the moment the elephant's head had hit the Serta Perfect Sleeper mattress, she was about to be awakened. "Be careful not to stand in front of her," warned Dr. Tuskectomy. "She can head-press you against the concrete block wall. You only need to see someone smashed into pasta one time to know that you have to be careful." The elephant was back on display the following day, enjoying good health and much more popularity among visitors with one tusk than she ever did with two.

When an animal is anesthetized for surgery, Marks and Neiffer simultaneously attempt to practice preventative medicine. The animal will be given a complete physical, including a dental inspection—and whatever else is necessary and/or possible, based upon time and resources. Because many of the animals on which they will work are priceless and endangered, and because boarded veterinary specialists are rare in areas of the country without veterinary schools, specialists from the world of human medicine are called in for support. Dentists Tom Brown and Mary Ann Anuszkiewicz have a typical family practice in an expanding suburb thirty minutes from the city line, but voluntary zoo work highlights their professional experiences. Photographs of the dentists in scrubs and gloves, posing with some of the animals they've treated, adorn their offices like diplomas.

In the van driving over to the primate facility, we all laugh and make faces as Neiffer explains that so far pus draining from the infected throat sac that is endangering Edna the orangutan's life had not presented serious drainage problems because Edna's mate, Julius, has been affectionately sucking it up and swallowing it in a misplaced act of love.

Minutes later, Don Neiffer loads his gun with a ketamine-powered dart and approaches Edna's cage. The rest of the team, including Marks, Karen, two anesthetists from a nearby women's hospital, Brown and Anuszkiewicz, two keepers, Lee Nesler, and I, huddle in the corner, out of sight, whispering. Fortunately, the process goes smoothly; Edna is soon nodding off.

The stretcher is like a chaise longue on wheels. Edna is belted down with bungee cords. As we roll her out of the primate house and into the waiting van, Lee Nesler looks down at Edna, a gigantic furry brown ball with a flat black nose and black fingernails, and croons. "She is beautiful; you've just got to love her, right?" As soon as the stretcher is lifted into the van and we all jump inside, a delivery truck pulls in front of us and stops. "Fellas," Lee Nesler yells out the window, "Move, please."

The driver is not paying attention, so Marks drives the van up on the sidewalk and goes around the truck. The sedative provides a twenty-five-minute window of opportunity for intubation and anesthesia. We don't want Edna waking up in the zoo hospital—or in this van—without being strapped down with something more substantial than bungee cords. Pound for pound, the orangutan is one of the most powerful species on Earth, reportedly capable of tearing apart the jaws of crocodiles that have attacked them. An orangutan at the zoo broke off a solid one-inch-thick iron bar from his holding cage. Orangutans are also priceless, with only about two thousand remaining in the wilds, exclusively in Sumatra and Borneo. After the hour-long procedure in which the tumor is removed and sutured, Marks, Nesler, and Neiffer clip Edna's toenails and fingernails, while the dentists examine and clean Edna's large yellow teeth. They discover an abscessed tooth—and pull it.

When we finally return Edna to her cage and lift her gently onto the straw-covered floor, everyone gathers around to watch her wake up. Lee Nesler and Don Neiffer lay their hands upon Edna, as if she is their little baby; together they comb her coat, cleaning off straw and debris, with Lee making reassuring cooing noises. Now everyone is talking quietly about the procedure; again we are experiencing that communal moment of peace, solitude, and satisfaction I have so frequently observed and described. We have worked very hard—and we all have other things to do. And yet, we linger here, waiting for Edna to wake. No one will leave until we know that she has emerged from the anesthesia.

Suddenly, Edna begins to cough and vomit fluid. Everyone is on their feet. The danger is regurgitation of food while being asleep, which is one of the reasons neither animals nor humans are permitted food prior to surgery. If Edna doesn't wake up—or if some action isn't taken in a hurry—she can die. The two anesthetists have placed the suction machine at the door of the cage, in preparation for this very complication. They rush to set it up and roll it into the cage, while Neiffer blots the fluid streaming out of Edna's mouth with a paper towel. They are just about ready to connect the machine when Lee Nesler sees Edna's eyes flicker. "Wait, here she comes." And then, speaking in a high voice on behalf of the orang, Lee imitates Edna. "Hi, you guys. Hi, hi, hi, what's happening?"

# FECALAS LIZARDAS—AND
# OTHER FUNNY JOKES

I find Don Neiffer sipping coffee in the tropical garden area of the National Aviary, one of two national, freestanding aviaries in the United States (the other is in Utah), where Marks and Neiffer share part-time veterinary responsibilities. At first light, the birds are feeding and therefore quite active. Standing quietly in shadow, we observe the aggressive mating ritual of the blue crowned pigeon. These are large birds of different shades of gray, and they're bumping into one another with humming grunts as they attempt to mate. I ask if there is a lot of aggression between the species at the aviary.

"Birds fight. Birds kill birds. Birds eat eggs." Neiffer pauses and shrugs. "On the other hand, South American birds know nothing about communication with birds from Africa, for example, but by and large, they do coexist quite well here." Birds are collected in relation to climate. An African lilac roller, which lives in the desert, for example, also would be included with an American desert roadrunner.

Neiffer seems frail and pale-looking at first sight, yet watching him function in the very vigorous capacity of a wildlife/zoo veterinarian, he is focused and energetic, although not as confident or as sure of himself as Marks. Graduating from the University of Pennsylvania in 1990, he first went into private practice, but found it to be a very unsatisfying experience. He volunteered at the zoo for nearly a year before being appointed associate veterinarian. His first and most challenging experience as a full-time zoo veterinarian actually took place at the National Aviary, involving reconstructive beak surgery for an endangered Southeast Asian bird, a great Indian hornbill. The bird flew into a wall and broke its lower mandible; an inoperative lower mandible meant slow starvation.

When eating, the hornbill grasps food with the end of its bill, tosses it up in the air, and then catches it in its mouth. Both mandibles must touch in order to manipulate the food. Six specialists, including Neiffer and Marks, a pediatric dentist, and a technician from a local dental lab, combined collective expertise to fashion an emergency replacement lower mandible for the bird. Constructed from state-of-the-art European dental acrylic similar to the orthodontic plastic used in retainers, the beak was matched so closely in color and shape and fit so carefully that it was difficult to recognize the artificial beak until Neiffer pointed out a few subtle discolorations.

As we watch the colorful bird feeding, Neiffer explains the hornbill's curious birthing ritual. A female goes into a hole in a tree. The male stays outside and muds up the hole so that no light gets in. He then pokes a hole through the mud, and spears food and transports it through the hole to the incubating mother, who consumes the nutrition for her babies. As each baby gets strong enough, they break through the mud, one by one, and then re-mud the hole to preserve the intimacy and darkness for the others. The mother will eventually leave, while the father will continue to feed the kids, and the process will go on until all of the chicks are out.

As we stroll leisurely through the complex, Neiffer repeatedly stresses the necessity of separating offspring from parents in zoos and in aviaries or shipping them to other facilities to safeguard against inbreeding. This is also why determining the sex of each animal or bird is so important and the reason he has been called in to work this morning—to surgically "sex" three scaley-naped pigeons, a process that often entails minor surgery. "I make an incision and go in to look for testes and ovaries," says Neiffer.

Jim Bonner, the veterinary technician in charge of the tiny aviary hospital, begins by putting a small empty syringe case attached to a small hose leading to a metal canister over the beak of the pigeon and turning on the gas. The little bird is instantly asleep. To intubate, a narrow plastic tube, which is connected to a tank of liquid anesthetic gas and oxygen, is inserted down the pigeon's trachea. A strip of adhesive is wrapped around the beak and tube so that the tube won't slip out of the trachea.

Neiffer, on his knees and bending over the table, turns the bird on its right side while Bonner holds the wings and the back feet down. With his finger, Neiffer literally begins to tear away the feathers on the left side—the paralumbar fossa—of the bird. Pigeons tend to lose a lot of body feathers easily as a defense against predators, but they grow back quickly. Working on the left side is important because female birds generally have only one ovary, which would be on the left. A male would have a testicle on each side.

Neiffer utilizes a scalpel to cut a hole through the skin, followed by a metal probe into the abdominal air sac. He spreads his hemostat to make the opening wider and then inserts the head of a sterile otoscope through the hole and attaches the otoscope, at which point he is able to view inside the bird. He peers into the otoscope as if he is peering into a microscope. There is a long pause as he manipulates the instrument, scratches his head, and grunts and groans before pronouncing: "It's a boy! White testicles. Big white testicles. Can't miss 'em." Bonner produces the second pigeon, and the process is repeated. After a while, Neiffer finally makes his pronouncement: "It's a boy."

"If they all turn out to be boys," Jim Bonner comments, "then you're going to have to explain why we keep getting more of these every year."

While we wait for a battery recharge on the otoscope so that the third pigeon can be sexed, Bonner brings in a hooded pita for a shipment exam. It's bound for the Memphis Zoo. "They have hooded pitas and we have banded pitas, except for this one hooded guy. We send them this hooded and receive a banded in trade." Neiffer examines the hooded pita quickly, gives him a manicure, both claws and the beak, as a going away present. Then Neiffer quickly sexes the third pigeon, also a boy.

"You haven't sexed a female pigeon since you've been working here," Bonner says.

The veterinarian's work is usually intense; Neiffer's ability to focus on his patients and hand-maneuver instruments within centimeters and millimeters rather than in inches is duly impressive, especially considering the labor-intensive, technologically limited tasks, such as sexing. At the same time, as Bonner and Neiffer repeatedly demonstrate, there's a fun-filled quality to the rhythm of their work. Usually, the banter between veterinarians, nurses, and technicians contains a surplus of scatological references, not surprising in an atmosphere where feces and urine are ever-present.

I once watched Neiffer and Marks work with Henry, an assistant curator; Ray, a reptile zookeeper; and Nancy, a fourth-year veterinary student at the zoo for a six-week externship, conduct a series of physicals on the zoo's crocodilian population—literally hundreds of them—at the outset, a seemingly impossible task. One after another, snakes and amphibians were lined up on an old plywood table located in the innards of the exhibit—the reptile pit—a space as dark, dank, and musty as an old cellar, with Neiffer working on one animal and Steve Marks working on another. Nancy was stationed at the counter beside the sink, across from the table, studying stool samples in a microscope and listening with amusement to their constant banter. They unroll a yellow tape, lay it over each reptile, and measure length in centimeters. Neiffer inserts a tube, pushes in liquid, then flushes it out slowly until the liquid turns brown.

Me: "What is that, Don?"

Don: "Fecalas lizardas."

Me: "Fecalas lizardas?"

Don: "Meaning," he smiles, "shit."

Across the table, a lizard won't keep its mouth open for Marks. He takes a credit card out of his wallet and jams the mouth open.

Nancy's examination of the fecalas lizardas under the microscope reveals worms, which means that all lizards, hundreds of them, must be treated.

Henry: "It's an hour and fifteen minutes, and we've only done three animals. You said we'd finish before lunch."

Steve: "I didn't say what day or which lunch."

With a long-handled hook, Henry lifts a crocodilian out of a fenced-in cage, offering it to Ray, who grabs it by the neck and tail and lays it on the glass. Both Henry and Ray must hold the crocodilian steady for Nancy, who listens and responds as Marks explains the proper technique by which she must insert her fin-ger into the anus to determine if the crocodilian is male or female.

Henry: "This will be the headline in *Animal Rights Magazine* next month: 'Male crocodilian violated by woman vet.'"

Next is a saltwater crocodile. Ray and Don dump him into a large plastic trash can in order to hold him on a scale, but he keeps trying to leap out. The thrashing of his tail against the wall of the can echoes like a drumbeat in the bowels of this building. His wriggling and jumping become so acute that they decide to put a lid over the top of the can. The alligator weighs twenty-nine pounds.

The bony scales on top of the crock are called "scoots," and the configuration of scales is unique—the best way in which the many similar species of crocodilians can be determined. Ray shows me the ear flaps, hard, stiff, and shell-like, which protect the ears and eyelids. The crocodilian is cool and surprisingly dry to the touch. His teeth are jagged like a small handsaw. Stom-achs of crocodilians are white and shiny like tile from a men's room floor.

There are steel doors on the back of this building, like jail doors, with windowpane-sized holes covered with thick metal webbing. Looking through these windows, you can see the red lights of the exhibit area outside, like the lights from a bordello. You can see families browsing in the dark, pointing at the ani-mals in the exhibit. But from this unique vantage point, the people look more curious than the animals, as if they are on display.

Ray: "Well, that's 11 animals down and 143 to go."

Abruptly, they quit for lunch.

# BABY-SITTING THE BONGO

Steven Marks is neither off-putting nor difficult to get along with, but he is very much the absentminded professor type; he doesn't try very hard to communicate or make people feel comfortable. The zoo hospital—the way it is set up—reflects Marks's personality in a certain way. It is organized, but devoid of a human element. There are no chairs for guests, no art on the walls. Marks seems to assume that humans and animals share similarly spare sensibilities.

His office itself is cold and cluttered, void of characteristic accoutrements. A photo of his wife and five-year-old son sits on the windowsill above his desk, along with another photo with his son in a backpack and with both father and son in cowboy safari hats. On his desk, there is a computer, a printer, and a telephone. He likes to use the speakerphone, another gesture toward impersonalization. Books and files are piled under his desk; he tosses papers on the floor when he's finished with them. I once watched him labor over the animal escape policy: He squinted at the computer screen, periodically sighing, pecking at the keyboard with two reluctant and awkward fingers. Once he looked up and asked me: "So how you spell thirty-ott six [30-06]?"

And yet, Marks is very much a romantic. For his tenth wedding anniversary (he married his high school sweetheart), he rented a tuxedo and surprised his wife, Kelly, by picking her up for dinner in a stretch limousine. He is not unaware of his problem relating to—and managing—people, which seems to be given minimal emphasis in veterinary school, but is of major importance in the outside world.

"Initially everything I did when I got my job here, I took to heart," he told me. "I was very rigid, arguing my point until I turned blue in the face; I'd argue with the keepers, the director, anybody who disagreed with me. It took me a long time to realize that there's more than one way to skin a goat; you can accomplish more by working with people and compromising on certain issues while not compromising your ethics than you can by refusing to give in."

I once witnessed a dispute between Marks and Lee Nesler having to do with a procedure that had been scheduled, which Nesler had attempted to cancel without informing Marks. Angry and nearly ranting to Don Neiffer about how inconsiderate his colleagues were, Marks decided to push on with the procedure because it had been scheduled—he had set aside the time—and he wanted it to be over and done with. Nesler was occupied with other animal-oriented matters in another part of the zoo, and so their debate was played out in cold tense tones for zoo personnel to hear on the walkie-talkies. But when Nesler finally arrived at the exhibit where the procedure was taking place, it was Marks who made peace. In five minutes they were joking around "like brother and sister," as Nesler had put it. That triggered a long and friendly discussion—a bonding experience about siblings and how disagreement, tension, and forgiveness brought friends and families closer. Nesler and Neiffer told me later that such compromise and understanding would never have happened with Marks just a year ago.

Although Marks is learning to work with people, his devotion to animals, especially those that are endangered, is legendary among his peers, as illustrated by his battle to save the life of a baby bongo, a large African antelope with a reddish brown coat, white stripes, and large floppy ears, with whom he became obsessed. It was born with a congenital defect that inhibited the function of its liver. Marks fought to keep it alive, but it became jaundiced, yellow in the eyes and skin. He called in a number of consultants, including a pediatrician and neonatologist from nearby Children's Hospital and a physician from the local blood bank because blood transfusions were required.

During the day, Marks could keep an eye on the bongo, but the fact that the bongo was alone at night drove him crazy. He worried about the possibility that the bongo would pull out the IV tube and bleed to death; he dreamed of arriving at the zoo hospital in the morning and discovering that the bongo was dead. That's why he began taking it home every night in the zoo van and set up IV feeding and antibiotic medications and a heat lamp to maintain a constant temperature in his kitchen. For a month, Marks slept on the couch downstairs, watching over the bongo, catnapping from time to time and jumping awake, crazed and frenetic, each time the infusion pump alarm went off.

As a last resort, after months of blood tests, fluid therapy, and tube and bottle-feeding, he arranged the back of the van in the same manner he had arranged his kitchen. An IV drip that led to an infusion pump was hung from the ceiling, and a bucket of syringes, antibiotics, tape, spare catheter, milk, and urine bucket were placed on the passenger seat, with the bongo in between. Then the animal was transported to the University of Pennsylvania's New Bolton Center, where it ended up in Wendy Vaala's NICU. But despite everyone's valiant efforts, it became perfectly clear that the bongo was gradually going downhill. The bongo's liver refused to function.

"At the end, we had it on a heated air mattress; they had a catheter in the bladder. We had two IV drips running, plus wires, monitors . . . it got really intensive. And the zoo put a nice financial effort towards it. You know, a bongo like that, a female, is worth $30,000. So you can justify a $4,000 bill at New Bolton in an effort to keep it alive. But Mother Nature still took her course. And the animal ended up dying."

As I sat with Marks that autumn afternoon in his office relating the painful story of the bongo's death, his lips began to tremble. He turned away, and we sat together in deep silence as he recomposed himself. The nurses in the NICU at New Bolton remember the dedication of the shy young veterinarian from the Pittsburgh Zoo and his sadness at the realization that the bongo could no longer survive. "He suffered," one nurse told me. "He—we all—got choked up."

But the turning point in Steve Marks's career actually had very little to do with his work with animals and very much to do with how he relates to and bonds with people. Last year, Marks suddenly realized that all his old friends and family were on the other side of the state, where he grew up. "You ask yourself, 'What's really important in life?'" He decided to resign from the zoo. He wrote the letter, turned it into the director, made the announcement during a staff meeting, and began cleaning the books from his shelf.

But throughout the following week, he began experiencing terrible misgivings—not because he thought he would miss the animals, not because of the loss of his terrific position at this very good zoo—but, surprisingly enough, because of the people and their startling emotional reaction to his announcement.

Steve Marks was embarrassed but not too surprised that Margie, the zoo secretary, had burst into tears when he had made his announcement, but he was totally taken aback by Don Neiffer's reaction. "Don was angry. He didn't lash out at me or anything, but he was very quiet and distant, just the way he had acted—kind of grieving—as when I told him the bongo died. I said, 'Why are you upset? You just got the job that you wanted so desperately. I waited until you got that job before I made this announcement.'

"Don told me, 'Because I wanted to learn from you.'

"And that totally set me back. I never thought of myself in that way, I mean as a teacher. I'm a doctor, an environmentalist. But Don said, 'The reason I came here was because you were here.' It made me realize that I was more than a veterinarian; I was a member of a community, a part of a family. I thought: 'It shouldn't be this painful to have to leave a job.' So, I asked the director if I could have my job back; thankfully, I got it."

Although his family and close friends are in another part of the state, Marks has come to realize that a special group of family and friends also surround him at the zoo—animal and human. He leads a unique veterinary lifestyle, a way of working and living—combining the outdoor life with the realities and complications of the city—to which most veterinarians aspire and only some actually achieve.

"I realized I needed to get out into the country again, which is where I grew up. And so we bought a farm." It is sixty-eight acres of timber and streams, with deer, grouse, wild turkey, and an abundance of plant life. "The land gives me relief and plea-sure. Weekends, I work with the chain saw, trying to clear the homesite. And it's like frontier land. Primitive, but rich and fertile. In retrospect, I'm very happy I decided to stay at the zoo."

Being a veterinarian, working with animals, sharing his love and devotion for animals with other like-minded people and becoming an integral part of a close-knit team, provides a good life. "The veterinary life is the one I will always want to live," Marks said.

# Icy

As I said at the beginning, I had been expecting to write a book about medicine, but I soon learned that medical science was only a part of what the veterinary world was all about. Veterinarians practice medicine and treat sick animals, but more than that and in a variety of crucial ways, veterinarians help people live more well-rounded, three-dimensional lives with animals as a primary balancing or anchoring factor.

Marks and Neiffer at the Pittsburgh Zoo are laboring for ecological reasons to preserve endangered species and to simultaneously bring pleasure and knowledge to people through interaction with exotic wild animals. The veterinarians at New Bolton love horses and derive pleasure from horses in a variety of ways. Certainly, experiences similar to Dr. Richardson's arthroscopic surgery procedure and the ongoing discomfort of the standardbred racehorse because of the financial investment of the owner are more common than anyone would like to admit, but less so than the abuses endured by human athletes in professional and NCAA-sanctioned college athletics. And the pleasure derived from owning a horse, competing with a horse—watching and wagering—is as satisfying to many fans as is soccer, basketball, and hockey.

Clearly, Gene Solomon and Paul Schwartz in Manhattan are working for people who own animals more so than the animals themselves. Some people, however, may question their motivations and intentions. Dining with a friend in Manhattan one evening and telling her about Pauline Wilson and her relationship with Gene Solomon, the friend became livid, repeatedly calling Gene Solomon a charlatan for taking Pauline's money. I attempted to defend Gene as best I could, but I soon realized I was fighting a losing battle. I listened to my friend rant and rave for a while and then changed the subject.

Initially, when I first learned about Pauline from Gene Solomon, I was intrigued because I thought her story might be amusing, perhaps even pitiful, and I did think Solomon's actions were suspect. But when I finally met Pauline and began to talk with her, my respect for her choices heightened because of her impressive and convincing commitment to preserve something she dearly loved; the fact that it was a cat seems almost irrelevant in her particular circumstances. Besides, it was not as if Pauline was denying herself or her family the basics of food and lodging to keep Baby Cat alive. The Wilsons were well-off and able to afford a fifty thousand dollar loss—at least this one time. And it was their money, not Medicaid money, nor HMO money; they had worked for what they owned and had the right to invest resources in their own way, no matter how eccentric some people might perceive it.

I once purchased a nearly new Porsche—a very expensive sports car I had coveted throughout my life—but when I finally fulfilled my dream, I discovered that it wielded considerably less satisfaction than I had expected. Recently, I took my son to Disney World. The first day at the Magic Kingdom, the first ride we chose was Peter Pan. The moment that the music started, the lights began flashing and we plunged into the darkened world of Never-Never Land, I burst into tears. Neither my son nor my wife knew that I was crying: That experience in the dark "Never-Never" with my family brought back haunting images of my past—and my needs as a very young boy for love, attention, and fun that went unfulfilled. Disney World was an expensive vacation and certainly not intellectually stimulating; some friends and colleagues scoffed at the waste of time and money. To me, it was an illuminating and defining moment of my life. The memories of this experience will linger forever with my son.

As I see it, Pauline's love for Baby Cat worked in a similar way. It might have been better for society as a whole for Pauline to have donated the fifty thousand dollars to the Salvation Army or even the Animal Rescue League, just as it might have been better for me and my son to have visited the Smithsonian Institution. But Pauline did not perceive such a responsibility. Her heart dictated her actions, which seems to be the only appropriate response.

As to the question of Baby Cat's suffering, about which my dinner companion had been so incensed? What about all the people in hospitals across the United States currently being kept alive on life support with no chance for survival and for whom our tax dollars pay much of the cost? What about heart transplants to infants whose chances of remaining alive to toddler age are minimal, at best? Rationalization only illustrates the ambivalence of such situations. I am not close enough to God to decide for other people when to make such significant decisions; neither is the friend with whom I had dinner that evening or anyone else I know.

* * *

Although Amy Attas described her mission as "God's Work," most veterinarians deny a higher calling; these are down-to-earth men and women who are basically attempting to make their living in a satisfying way with animals—and people. But the fact is, veterinarians will often treat patients more like God's Children than their human doctor counterparts. One might be tempted to say that it is easier to treat animals as innocents, but while probably true, this logic will never justify an MD's dehumanizing behavior to patients and their families. Nor will it diminish the humanistic way in which veterinarians do their work.

Veterinarians also possess privileges that are currently out of the realm of possibility for human doctors, foremost among which is euthanasia. In fact, it was this very compassionate act of putting a suffering animal to death that eventually helped me select the veterinary life as a book topic.

Icy was a mostly black smallish German shepherd with frosty white trimmings I had raised from a tiny puppy. He spent the days with me in my office as I wrote. When my first wife and I were divorced, however, Icy, whom I had obedience-trained and who had been awarded many blue ribbons for excellence in obedience trials, went over the edge, becoming unpredictable and often hostile to strangers. Once, sitting at my side on the street as I talked with a friend, he suddenly leaped at her four-year-old son and lifted a chunk of skin from the fleshy part of his cheek directly below his eyes. A quarter-inch upward, and the boy could have been blinded.

Friends urged me to put Icy to sleep, insisting that a dog exhibiting such frightening and hostile behavior has crossed over a line of oblivion from which for an animal there is usually no return. But I held on to Icy for months, despite his attack and his hostile threatening behavior to other guests. My personal situation was pretty dismal, and Icy was not only my best friend, but the last vestige of my six-year marriage, a symbol and a loving connection I did not want to release. But the day I found him chewing on the ankle of a friend who had come to visit and saw the surprise and terror in my friend's eyes, I realized that enough was enough.

I contacted the captain of the local police K-9 corps, who, accompanied by a young officer in search of a canine partner, arrived at my house the following afternoon. They watched through the kitchen window while I took Icy out into the backyard and put him through his paces. It was a perfect performance. Icy would sit, heel, lie down, fetch, and come in response to either voice commands or hand signals. After a while, the captain came out onto the back porch: "Yes, we'll take him," he said. "But we want him right now."

"I hadn't planned on giving him up so soon," I said, panicking. "I just wanted you to meet him."

"In our experience in these cases, the best thing is for us to take your dog away before you think too much about it."

This advice seemed logical. And I couldn't think of an alternative solution. I handed the leash to the young officer, turned my back, and walked to the front window to watch them depart. My last memory of Icy was when he paused at the back of the police van and turned toward me with a look of surprise and abandonment I will never forget, as if to say, "You are letting them take me away? How could you?" I knew that my answer was "How could I not?"

Some months after Icy's departure in the K-9 van, I received a phone call from the secretary of the precinct to which Icy and his police officer partner had been assigned. She explained that Icy had attacked the officer's children (K-9 dogs will usually live at home with their human partners) and had become increasingly unreliable. Tomorrow morning the officer was driving him to the country to be introduced to an elderly man on a small farm, where he might find a home as a guard dog. If the man was not interested, Icy would be euthanized. She was calling to say that I could have Icy back if I wanted, however, and subsequently make the decision about Icy's fate on my own.

I missed Icy, would have enjoyed having him back—the old Icy, that is—and I felt somewhat responsible for the change in his nature. But my guilt for what happened was not reason enough to bring this angry dog who hurt little children back to my new home. I could not, on the other hand, let Icy go without one last look. The following morning I got up early, drove to the police officer's house to wait surreptitiously for him to transport Icy to the country. I caught sight of him in his family car with Icy sitting in the backseat peering out of the rear window. I instinctively began to follow.

About forty minutes later, the officer turned off the highway onto a narrow, isolated blacktop road and then pulled into a dirt driveway in front of a small frame farmhouse. I drove to the top of a hill where I could watch the comings and goings at the house while the officer led Icy on a leash onto the porch. I finally caught a clear glimpse of Icy, who seemed a bit more filled out than I remembered him, but fit and healthy. The old man was short, skinny, and scraggly. The police officer did most of the talking, periodically pointing down at Icy and petting him, with the old man nodding warily. It wasn't hard to know, judging by their body language, that the conversation was not going in Icy's favor. Within a few minutes, the visit was over. The two men shook hands cursorily.

The officer then drove into a nearby town, down the main street, turning off onto a side road and stopping in front of a small veterinary hospital. In retrospect, I should have known exactly what was happening as soon as Icy and the police officer stopped at the veterinarian's office, but I sat in my car across the street, theorizing that the farmer had insisted that Icy undergo a physical examination before accepting him on the farm. I didn't become fully aware that something else was happening until the police officer emerged from the veterinarian's office, got into his car, and drove away—alone.

I jumped out of my car and dashed into the veterinary office. An elderly woman at a small reception desk looked up and smiled. I asked to see the doctor. Before she could answer, I could hear in the background Icy's unmistakable bark—but not the friendly barking I remembered so clearly as he excitedly greeted me each time I came home, a happy welcome I would never forget. The tone and timbre were different; it was an angry, snarling sound. The woman informed me that the doctor was busy. I said that I would come back later. I left the office and followed the sound to the rear of the building and peeked inside an open window.

For an instant I saw Icy, my same wonderful beautiful black dog with the frosted paws and eyebrows, but a glimpse into his angry, frantic eyes convinced me that he was also very different from the dog I loved. Something had happened to Icy over those months with the K-9 corps—the beginnings of which I had witnessed prior to his departure from my life. He had lost his center, his stability, his awareness of right and wrong.

Veterinarians lack a basic understanding of how and why this condition in animals comes about, but it is almost always disseminated by thoughtless and one-dimensional breeding practices. Too much emphasis is placed on physical conformity by owners and breeders at the expense of temperament, thereby perpetuating unsound mental traits in certain breeds of dogs. At the same time, the entire breed can suffer great prejudice, such as in the case of German shepherds, although the vast majority possesses a basically harmless temperament. The aggression displayed by these dogs is often fear-related, sparked by cruelty and mistreatment. Mental or behavioral disturbances suffered by animals are probably not dissimilar to the quirks in the human mind that cause a perfectly settled and sane man or woman to suddenly, without a clear and discernible reason, lose touch with reality.

When this happens, we cannot euthanize human beings, but because in this society animals are subservient to humans and considered to be their property, owners possess the right of disposal. Veterinarians consider euthanization both a burden and a great luxury, in that they possess the capability of saving a patient (and family) from prolonged agony and pain. I didn't like the idea of euthanizing Icy, which is exactly what the veterinarian was in the process of doing, but in retrospect, I think I understood it.

The veterinarian was an older man, perhaps in his late sixties, slender and balding, and had obviously performed this very same act of mercy hundreds of times. He approached Icy with a quiet tenderness and a soothing, sensitive voice that calmed the angry dog. His tenderness calmed me, too. Icy sniffed at the veterinarian's fingers before permitting the man to pet him gently and soothingly. Icy began to whimper. I don't think he was aware of what was about to happen to him, but I do imagine that he felt a momentary sense of rest. The hypodermic needle suddenly appeared in the veterinarian's hand, and almost immediately, Icy slipped soundlessly to the linoleum.

Animal euthanasia is often difficult for human beings to accept because people tend to be very anthropomorphic about animals and to assume that the threat and loss of life means the same thing to an animal as to a human being. People who know animals will tell you that animals experience fear and pain, just like humans, and they will display the same general range of symptoms as a human would show in similar physical circumstances. But they don't worry about losing their lives, and they do not fear or conceive of death. At that point at which the euthanasia occurs, animals close their eyes and go to sleep as they do every day or night, without a preconceived notion or expectation of waking up the following morning.

This is one of the reasons veterinarians are veterinarians: Animals are so much more accepting than people and consequently are often so very responsive to the work of a veterinarian. Even when animals are vicious, veterinarians don't often display animosity. "You don't hate the animal," Amy Attas told me, "you simply fear it. And you know that they're hostile or aggressive for a reason. And the reasons are usually better than human reasons. Animals do not display racial prejudice; they don't have ulterior motives. It's always a functional thing. If they are being vicious to us, it's because they're afraid and they're trying to protect themselves or their owners. This is a quality to admire."

The playwright Eugene O'Neill was an avid animal lover who treated his pets with the kindness and regard of people, but also understood that dogs and cats were significantly different from human beings. In a story entitled "The Last Will and Testament of an Extremely Distinguished Dog," O'Neill wrote:

Dogs do not fear death as men do. We accept it as part of life, not as something alien and terrible which destroys life. What may come after death, who knows? I would like to believe . . . that there is a Paradise where one is always young and full-bladdered; where all the day one dillies and dallies with a continuous multitude of houris, beautifully spotted; where jack rabbits that run fast but not too fast (like the houris) are as the sands of the desert; where each blissful hour is mealtime; where in long evenings there are a million fireplaces with logs forever burning, and one curls himself up and blinks into the flames and nods and dreams, remembering the old brave days on earth, and the love of one's Master and Mistress.

O'Neill's empathy helped me understand and accept what Icy might next experience, although at the time of this incident, I was nearly overwhelmed with a surge of remorse and guilt that had almost triggered a daring intervention; my momentary fantasy was to dive through the window, scoop Icy off the floor a split second prior to the injection, and run away with him. But I had realized that the damage had been done long before; Icy and I could not live happily ever after. A rescue would simply complicate my life and mislead Icy. He would have to be put to sleep eventually.

When I returned home later that day, I sat down in the room I used as an office. A photo of Icy, his white-tipped paw resting on his favorite toy, a basketball, which he had endlessly pushed and chased around our backyard, was above my desk. I sat for a while and thought about the fun I had had with Icy and the loyalty he had displayed through all of our years together. Before leaving the room, I kissed his photograph and turned out the light. My lingering memory of Icy's death is very positive, which is partially because of the dignified way in which that elderly veterinarian treated my dog. Of all of the services veterinarians provide, I appreciate and respect euthanasia the most. Not that one could view the taking of a life as a positive quality, but in all of the cases I observed, veterinarians were compassionate and respectful during euthanasia. Each had his or her own manner and technique, but their actions always involved touching—the laying of their hands on the animal, gently and with dignity. In these moments, I sensed the weight of pain and suffering they shouldered—true empathy for animals and their owners. Each time they knelt to put an animal to sleep, I sensed a profound sorrow, as if something of substance also died inside the veterinarian. But these men and women were fulfilling their responsibility as doctors and humanitarians, a basically unacknowledged act in an unspoken art.

# INDEX